THE NATURAL WAY SERIES

Increasing numbers of people worldwide are
falling victim to illnesses which modern medicine,
for all its technical advances, often seems
powerless to prevent – and sometimes actually
causes. To find cures for these so-called 'diseases
of civilization' more and more people are turning
to 'natural' medicine for an answer. *The Natural
Way* series aims to offer clear, practical and
reliable guidance to the safest, gentlest and most
effective treatments available – and so to give
sufferers and their families the information they
need to make their own choices about the most
suitable treatments.

THE NATURAL WAY WITH

Migraine

Eileen Herzberg

Approved by the
**AMERICAN HOLISTIC MEDICAL ASSOCIATION
& BRITISH HOLISTIC MEDICAL ASSOCIATION**

Series medical consultants
Dr Peter Albright MD & Dr David Peters MD

Series editor
Richard Thomas

E L E M E N T
Shaftesbury, Dorset ● Rockport, Massachusetts
Brisbane, Queensland

© Eileen Herzberg 1994

First published in Great Britain in 1994 by
Element Books Limited
Shaftesbury, Dorset SP7 8BP

Published in the USA in 1994 by
Element Books, Inc.
PO Box 830, Rockport, MA 01966

Published in Australia in 1994 by
Element Books Limited for
Jacaranda Wiley Limited
33 Park Road, Milton, Brisbane 4064

Reprinted 1995

Cover design by Max Fairbrother
Designed and typeset by Linda Reed and Joss Nizan
Printed and bound in Great Britain by
BPC Paperbacks Limited

British Library Cataloguing in Publication
data available

Library of Congress Cataloging in Publication
data available

ISBN 1–85230–495–2

Contents

List of Illustrations

Dedication

Dedicated to everyone who wants to
say goodbye to their migraine

Acknowledgements

I would particularly like to thank Jessica Macbeth for support, encouragement, healing and inspiration over and beyond anything I could have dared to ask for. I am also grateful to Dr Roger Lichy who fed me food, facts and affection and to Lucy who behaved herself so wonderfully (Lucy is the faithful LCII Applemac who only crashed once during the whole book!).

More thanks go to everyone at the Penzance Natural Health Centre, Bruce Matheson at the Truro Natural Health Centre, to Jo Liddell at the British Migraine Association, Simon Lichtenstein and to all the other practitioners and people who made this book possible.

Introduction

'That no one dies of migraine seems to someone deep into an attack an ambiguous blessing'
- Joan Didion, *The White Album* (Penguin, 1968)

Princess Margaret gets them, so does Princess Diana, President Ulysses S Grant had them and so do butchers, bakers and candlestick-makers. Migraine strikes people in all walks of life everywhere, in primitive tribal societies as well as sophisticated civilized ones. Estimates vary but this devastating complaint afflicts an estimated one in ten of the population, although some say it may be as high as one in five.

Although only about a third of those who suffer with migraine go to their doctors for it this book is for all migraine-sufferers. It describes the various drugs that doctors prescribe – and how they work (or not), how you can help yourself and how natural therapists can help. Natural therapy here is used in the widest possible sense, meaning any form of treatment that doesn't involve drugs. The book is also full of stories of people who have had migraine. Notice the past tense. They've got rid of their migraines. Maybe this book will also help you to say 'goodbye' to yours.

Eileen Herzberg
Penzance
England

CHAPTER 1

What is migraine?

All about its symptoms and causes

'It's a blinding, sharp, jabbing pain which affects my vision which goes blurry and sparkly and my balance goes, my co-ordination goes, I can't see, I'm focused on the pain, it's difficult to grip cups, the pain claws all energy to one part of the body. I feel nauseous and have to lie down in a darkened room and drink lots of fluids. I think I'm dying of a brain tumour.' – MARK P.

'I get such a splitting headache, I can't describe the pain. I often get visual disturbances, a bit like an acid trip where the focal point is split into a kaleidoscope. It moves around all the time, it's a prism that's broken up into colours of the rainbow. It's very pretty but I feel disconnected, I can't concentrate and the back of my head is a slow deadening feeling and it's very difficult to concentrate.' – SUE M.

'The day before I get a surge of energy and it starts with a slight headache and then it gets much worse – sometimes I get the lights, sometimes the vomiting, my words come out backwards before an attack.' – SUSAN B.

'At first my hearing would become extremely clear and it was as if I was looking at things from another level, from a long way away, like an out-of-body

experience. It was very clear. Then I would start seeing zig-zag patterns of lights. Then I would get very
ill, with nausea and headaches. I would feel better if
I could make myself sick.' – FREEDA G.

'The pain was so bad I thought that if only I could
gouge out my eye, the pain might go away. I was
nauseous but I couldn't vomit. I wished I could be
sick to get rid of the nausea.' – MARION G.

There is nothing easy or straightforward about migraine.
As the above cases illustrate, nothing about migraine or
migraine-sufferers is true for everyone. Each person's
migraine is as unique as his or her fingerprints. Some
people's migraines can be caused by sleeping too long,
yet others by too much exercise. Some people can avert a
migraine by lying quietly in a darkened room, others can
take evasive action by vigorous exercise.

A migraine is much more than just a bad headache. In
fact you might not get a headache at all – even though
the *Concise Oxford Dictionary* defines migraine as a
'recurrent, paroxysmal headache often with nausea and
disturbance of vision'. Many doctors say that a migraine
must be accompanied by disturbances of vision or of the
stomach and intestines.

Equally, you may have a bad headache that is not a
migraine. If the headache is short and sharp it might be a
cluster headache (see box). If the headache is almost continuous then it might be a tension headache – or you
may be taking too much medication (see p. 21).

Many people describe a full-blown migraine, which
may last two hours to seventy-two hours, as a sick
headache or bilious attack because of the nausea and
vomiting that goes with the headache. Others only suffer
from the nausea and vomiting and don't get the
headaches.

Some people experience visual disturbances before an

attack. These are known as 'auras' and might consist of bright lights around objects or partial or full loss of vision. For example, if you are reading you might see a hole in the print. Some people lose half of their visual field. Some people only suffer from these auras – and don't get headaches or nausea and vomiting. During migraine most people are hypersensitive to light and noise.

Different sorts of migraine and headaches

Migraine without aura
As this is experienced by so many people it used to be called 'common migraine'.

Migraine with aura
The aura lasts about half an hour and is usually followed by the other migraine symptoms – but it may not. This type of migraine is also known as 'classical migraine'.

Migraine without headache
As you would expect, this is where the aura is present but not the headache. It used to be called 'migraine equivalents'.

Status migrainosus
A prolonged migraine attack in which the headache may change in intensity but never really disappears.

Cluster headaches
The attacks come in clusters of 6-12 weeks, often at the same time of the year. The headache itself is usually short (30 minutes to two hours) but there may be several a day. Cluster headaches used to be called 'migrainous neuralgia'. They are not really migraines at all and are quite rare. They are also sometimes called an 'alarm headache', because they wake you in the morning with a severe pain behind one eye (always the same eye), the eye goes red, tears may stream from it and the nostril on the same side will either be blocked or discharge a clear fluid. The pain is so bad that you may have to pace the room or clutch your head and some-women say they'd rather have another baby than the pain.

Tension type headaches
These can be continual or can come back at the same time every day. They can last from half an hour to a week. They are often described as being like a tight band right round the skull or as pressure on top or the sides of the head. About 80 per cent of people have experienced tension headache, which often starts in the neck and spreads up to the head. Tension headaches don't make you vomit but can cause mild nausea. Also they don't usually cause sensitivity to light, sound or movement.

Drug-associated headaches
Too many painkillers or ergotamine-based medication can cause daily headaches. Many other drugs can also have headaches as a side-effect.

How to know if you've got a migraine

With all these different varieties of headache how do you know you've got a migraine? The only person who can make an accurate diagnosis is someone who is medically-qualified – however, you can make an intelligent guess. Although people experience migraine in many different ways the pattern is always the same:

- a warning signal such as anxiety or lethargy, followed by
- violent headache
- and/or nausea
- and/or vomiting
- extreme sensitivity to light, sound, movement
- lasting two hours to 72 hours
- normal health between attacks.

One of the most common aspects of migraine is that you'll probably get some warning that it's coming. Even if you don't have auras you may experience some tell-tale signal that tells you a migraine is coming. This is known as a 'prodrome' and it can assume almost any form. Some people complain of a terrible lethargy before the migraine. Yet others experience a sudden surge of energy. For example, the famous migraine-sufferer the Victorian novelist George Eliot complained of feeling 'dangerously well' before a migraine.

'When a really bad one is coming, I start to lisp, my tongue doesn't function properly, and my boss says it's time to go home and go to bed. He knows that if I wait I won't be able to drive' is how one woman described her warning sign. Other warning signs include some startling contrasts:

- water-retention or thirst
- hyperactivity or yawning and lethargy
- anxiety or euphoria
- numbness or hypersensitivity
- hunger or loss of appetite
- diarrhoea or constipation
- difficulty speaking (dysphasia) or unusually articulate
- dullness or unusually witty
- muddle-headedness or unusually clear-thinking

A word of advice: If you think none of this applies to you ask the people closest to you – can they tell when you're about to get a migraine?

Migraine 'auras'

Migraine 'auras' can be loosely defined as hallucinations. They can affect any of the senses – sight, smell, hearing, taste or touch – or can show as an alteration of consciousness. Some people experience auras as purely visual, others experience them as a distortion of reality. These reality distortions can be so disturbing that people don't like to talk about them, so they may be more com mon than is generally realized. Auras can be positive as well as negative:

A positive aura consists of bright lights, zig zags and patterns. Or it can affect one of the other senses so that, for example, you hear music that isn't there.

A negative aura, on the other hand, is when there is something missing. For example, if someone sees a head but no face, or a hole develops in what they are reading. Or it can affect one of the other senses, so that, for example, you can't hear people talking, or lose your sense of smell or taste.

Visual auras (also known as *scotoma*) can consist of stars, bright lights, swirling patterns or even elves. The aura can be quite complicated, like a Persian carpet, or complete scenes or divine visions of people, animals and birds. Everything may seem suddenly very small – or very large (we've probably got migraine auras to thank for Lewis Carroll's *Alice Through the Looking Glass*).

Hallucinatory smells can be extremely pleasant – like flowers – or extremely unpleasant and distasteful.

Hallucinatory sounds can take the form of music or noise and hearing can be very acute – or sounds can become very indistinct, as if they were coming from a long way away.

Hallucinatory feelings can take the form of extreme sensitivity to touch, a temporary weakness in one half of the body, a change in muscle tone (either extremely tense or complete loss of muscle tone), or a change in sense of taste (some people get a strange taste in their mouth, others lose their sense of taste altogether).

Hallucinatory states of consciousness can take the form of a complete change in memory, speech, or perception.

The aura stage can last for a few minutes or as long as an

hour and this is usually followed by the other symptoms of headache, nausea and vomiting, and sensitivity to light and/or sound. There may be a gap between the aura ending and the headache starting. Some people only suffer the aura sensation and no headache.

Migraine headache symptoms

The headache may start as a normal headache and then increases in severity, becoming a throbbing pain, which is made worse by movement, light or noise. It's usually a one-sided headache, although sometimes it's the whole head that hurts.

Some people complain that it feels as if their head is bursting and they may be right. A woman who had a part of her skull removed was observed during a migraine. Her brain literally bulged outwards. At the height of the attack it stopped pulsating, then she would vomit and sleep, and the tense brain would revert to its normal slackness.

Nausea, vomiting, dizziness or sensitivity to light and sound may accompany the headache.

The end of the attack

Some people find that the only way to end an attack is to sleep it off, although this may be impossible until the migraine has subsided. Many people say that after a migraine they experience particularly long, deep and refreshing sleeps.

Others find that the migraine only ends when they can arouse themselves in some way, and it is this arousal that gets rid of the migraine. This can take the form of hiccuping or belching or even voracious eating. Even sudden mental or physical exercise like making love, arm-wrestling – anything to get the adrenalin going –

can bring an attack to an end or even avert an attack altogether.

Some people find that their migraine ends with some form of release. This may take the form of crying, vomiting, urinating, sweating, sneezing, a nosebleed or the start of menstruation.

After the attack

You may feel totally washed-out or refreshed and euphoric. The feeling of euphoria is more likely after menstrual migraine, less likely if you've experienced vomiting or diarrhoea.

Between attacks

You may feel so well in between migraines that you don't consult your doctor. If you only have a migraine once a year it is very easy to shrug it off and do nothing about it. But if you get frequent, severe migraine it can be so devastating that it can seriously affect the quality of your life.

CHAPTER 2

Causes and 'triggers'

Who migraine affects and how it can be set off

Migraine is no respector of fame or fortune. Famous 'migraineurs' include St Paul, Julius Caesar, Charles Darwin, Immanuel Kant, Lewis Carroll, President Ulysses S Grant, Sigmund Freud, Princess Margaret, and Princess Diana. Edgar Allan Poe had such excruciating migraines that he sometimes rushed outside to bury his head in snow.

Migraine has been recognized and written about since the times of ancient Egypt, and Moses might have been suffering from a migraine aura when he saw the burning bush or the pillar of fire. Even after all this time we still don't know why so many millions of people suffer from it. It seems to run in families – six out of ten sufferers have a close family member who also has migraine.

But it doesn't *always* run in families and no one has identified a migraine 'gene'. However, women seem to suffer more than men. Only 30 per cent of people with migraine are men but this might be an under-estimate. Men may simply be more reluctant to admit to migraines than women.

Research suggests that migraine sufferers are no more intelligent or more sensitive than non-sufferers and we're left with no clear idea of why some people should get migraine and others don't. The people who get migraine have different personalities and temperaments, sizes and ages. Very young children and even babies can get migraine and it can continue right up to old age.

People who get migraine may be able to cope with just as much stress as non-sufferers, but their reactions are different. People react to stress in many different ways: stress is blamed for asthma, psoriasis, arthritis, hypertension, ulcers – and of course headaches and migraine. What makes migraine sufferers different from other people?

The latest research shows that people who have had what are known as 'out-of-body experiences' are more than twice as likely to be migraine sufferers than a control group. An out-of-body experience is where people have the sensation of leaving the physical body for a short time. This fits in neatly with one theory which states that migraine is caused by some kind of 'short circuitry' in the brain.

Is migraine the brain short-circuiting?

The Victorians recognized migraine as 'nerve storms' and in his book *Migraine* Oliver Sacks describes them as 'epilepsy in slow motion'. Brainwaves can be measured – and there is sometimes a similarity between what happens during a migraine aura and an epileptic attack. An electroencephalogy (or EEG) machine can measure brainwave patterns through electrodes in the scalp. On a graph these measurements can look like sharp spokes when someone is having an epileptic fit – and it can sometimes (but not always) show a similar pattern when someone is having a migraine aura. Irregular brainwave patterns have also been noticed in some people who suffer from migraine, even when they are migraine-free.

People who have had out-of-body experiences are also more likely to have hypomania – the ability to experience heightened excitement or arousal. People who tend to be placid and phlegmatic tend not to have out-of-body experiences – and may be less likely to get migraine. Dr Charles McCreery, the research officer at the Institute of Psychophysical Research in Oxford, says that the link between out-of-body experiences, hypomania and migraine is quite logical: 'Migraine is very much a disorder of arousal. It starts with this period of hyper-excitement or a sense of tremendous well-being, then comes the pain, you go into the slump and then you come out of it.'

It may be that people who have migraine don't filter sensations very effectively. There is a primitive part of the brain known as the reticular activating system (RAS) which mainly signals alarm or calm (see 'All about the brain' on page 14). Some people have a wide open RAS that lets in a lot of information, others have an RAS which lets in less information – and this could also explain why some people have a tendency towards migraine, and others don't .

What brings on a migraine?

'I love the people with their simple straightforward minds. It's only that their smell brings on my migraine' – Bertolt Brecht

Anything that can cause an ordinary headache can bring on a migraine. Common causes of both ordinary headaches and migraines include: too much sleep, too little sleep, stress, high altitude, low blood-sugar, tobacco, alcohol, withdrawal symptoms from caffeine and other drugs, and certain types of foods (see box 'Suspect foods' on page 46).

It's often a combination of factors that brings on a migraine. Moreover it's often when you are feeling stressed, tired and most vulnerable that you are most likely to eat and drink the very things that will bring on a migraine.

'I found I was more likely to get a migraine if I was under terrific strain,' is how the British novelist Jean Stubbs describes it. 'I discovered that four things all together brought on a migraine and it was the combination that did it. If I had cheese, red wine, coffee and chocolate I knew I'd be for it. I couldn't seem to avoid that combination. It would happen by accident, particularly when I was having lunch with my publisher.'

All about the brain

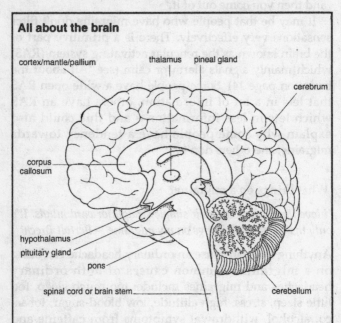

Fig. 1 The human brain

In evolutionary terms, the oldest part of the brain is the reptilian brain, also known as the brain stem which controls basic life-saving functions such as breathing, heart regulation and blood circulation. It also monitors and regulates all our muscular activity and sensory perceptions. The reptilian brain includes the reticular activating system (RAS), a sort of volume control of sensations. People whose reticular activating system filters out a great deal of information must give themselves lots of stimulation to feel alive. They will tend to be extroverts and may turn to stimulants. On the other hand, someone who has an open RAS which admits large quantities of information and sensations to awareness will not want additional stimulation and will tend to be introverts. We recognize these people as being sensitive, and they may even try to lower the stimulation they receive by drinking alcohol or taking other depressant drugs. We don't yet know if there is a relationship between introverts, an open RAS and migraine.

The RAS makes sure we pay attention to the new and potentially dangerous, but allows us to ignore what is familiar and safe. It signals stress or relaxation, sending signals of calm, alarm, or no change to the mammalian brain which is situated just above the reptilian brain. The mammalian brain, or limbic system, is responsible for our instinctive animal emotions such as rage, fear, panic, pleasure and grief, as well as altered states of consciousness such as euphoria and bliss. The limbic system is controlled by the hypothalamus, nicknamed the 'brain's brain', which links the body and emotions, controlling the body's internal organs and regulating its response to pleasure and pain.

All sensory information from the outside world is delivered to the hypothalamus: if the information is interpreted as stressful the hypothalamus releases chemicals that cause glands such as the pituitary and adrenals to release stress hormones into the bloodstream, resulting in the 'fight or flight response'. The hypothalamus responds to the absence of sensations by inhibiting the release of stress hormones and increasing the secretion of neurochemicals such as endorphins, producing the state of relaxation. The hypothalamus has the highest concentration of serotonin in the nervous system. We don't know much about migraine, but we do know that it has something to do with serotonin.

How the brain can play tricks: Reality distortion

'Words mean nothing to me and I cannot picture what's been described to me. I have been told that

Jackie has phoned and I think that I don't know anyone of that name. But after the migraine I know that
Jackie is my sister.' – SUE HARLOW.

'I didn't think I had migraine, I thought I was going
mad. The visual disturbance was very frightening,
flashing lights and then everything went like a photo-
graph torn in four' – FRANCES .

One of the extraordinary things about migraine is that it dis-
torts our perception of reality. Some descriptions of migraine
auras sound like LSD trips – and there does seem to be a
relationship between what LSD does to the brain and what
people experience when they have a migraine.

Most people think that our senses tell the brain what's real
and what isn't. But American psychologist Ronald Melzack
suggests the brain has its own sense of reality our senses
merely modify. This may explain why the brain conjures up
phantom limbs after they have been amputated. Melzack
calls this inherent state of reality the 'fundamental neuro-sig-
nature' of the brain. This is the brain's signature before we
are born and may be one explanation why some people suffer from migraines and others don't.

We experience this same primordial (pre-birth) brainwave
state in deep meditation and the same state can be experienced in a flotation tank, an enclosed chamber in which you
float in shallow salt-water. The sensory deprivation of floating in a warm, dark environment produces profound relaxation, a deeply meditative state said to be similar to the
pre-birth state.

How the brain senses pain: the 'Gate' theory

The 'Gate' theory of pain was first proposed by psychologist
Ronald Melzack and anatomist Patrick Wall in 1965. They
suggested that pain messages only reach the brain when
the nervous system opens the pain gate. Pleasure rushes to
the brain quicker than pain, so that messages of pleasure,
such as warmth, may close the gate on pain, such as
headache.

Pain gates open with:
- depression
- hopelessness

Pain gates close with:
- warmth
- enjoyment
- hope

This theory may explain why migraine pain varies in intensity from person to person and from one attack to another and during different times in a person's life.

The causes of migraine

'Migraine is essentially a derangement of the nerve cells of the brain.' – W R Gowers

Scientists used to believe that migraine was caused by the blood vessels going into the brain narrowing and then expanding. In other words those pounding headaches are literally caused by too much blood flooding the brain. But this begs the question: what tells the blood vessels to contract and expand?

Scientists now think that serotonin holds an important key because drugs that often help migraine also affect serotonin levels. What is serotonin? Serotonin is a *neurotransmitter*. A neurotransmitter is a chemical 'messenger'. It is released where two nerve cells meet, allowing or preventing electrical impulses to pass from one nerve cell to another.

Serotonin is only a means of communication. It is the nerves themselves that do the work. Depending on which nerve cells are communicating with each other, this can affect sleep patterns, mood, pain perception, temperature regulation, appetite, heart and circulation. When serotonin is released, blood vessels contract. As serotonin levels fall, the blood vessels dilate. Serotonin levels are high before a migraine, low afterwards.

Hunger, fatigue, stress, food, lighting and drugs can all affect serotonin levels.

Serotonin levels can fall as a result of:
- stress
- low blood sugar

Serotonin levels can rise as a result of:
- oxygen
- vomiting
- foods containing 'amines' such as cheese, chocolate and oranges
- foods containing the amino acid tryptophan such as milk and turkey. (Tryptophan is transported to the brain by insulin where it is converted into serotonin).

Serotonin is also affected by hormones: an *increase* in the 'female' hormone oestrogen triggers an increase in serotonin. The birth-control pill containing oestrogen produces headaches in some women when serotonin levels fall in the pill-free days when the body is not receiving extra oestrogen (and, hence, extra serotonin). A *drop* in oestrogen levels during menstruation produces a decrease in serotonin, which can thus bring on a migraine as the blood vessels dilate.

Serotonin binds with the hallucinatory drug LSD (*lysergic acid diethylamide*) and some of the drugs that are used in the treatment of migraine come from the LSD family. For example, *ergotamine* is based on lysergic acid and so is *methysergide*. Drug therapy relies on the way certain chemicals affect serotonin production and in the next chapter we'll look at how various drugs affect serotonin production and the way blood vessels contract and dilate.

CHAPTER 3

Conventional treatments and approaches

What your doctor is likely to say and do

'My doctor just prescribed tranquillizers – and I
said, thanks, but no thanks and walked out the
door.'

'My doctor said that he would prescribe anything I
thought might help. He also suggested I join the
Migraine Association.'

'My neurologist said I should learn how to meditate.'

How doctors react to migraine depends on their own
personality, prejudices and experiences. If they happen
to suffer from migraine themselves their attitudes may
be sympathetic – but they may also take the view that
they haven't found anything that could actually cure
migraine so why should your experience be any different?

If your migraine has begun recently and you are worried that it may be something more sinister – like a brain
tumour, for example – ask for a brain scan. If the doctor
points out that most migraines are nothing to worry
about tell him or her you would still like to be checked,
just to put your mind at rest. Don't be afraid to be
assertive.

If you don't get migraines very often the doctor may

prescribe a pain-killer, a serotonin antagonist or ergotamine to constrict your blood vessels.

If your migraines are frequent your doctor may start you on long-term preventive treatment that will consist of a daily dose of a beta-blocker, *pizotifen*, calcium-blocker or some other form of treatment such as anti-depressants to control serotonin production.

Treatment is usually a case of trial-and-error. If your medication is not effective or you are having side-effects ask your doctor to change your treatment. If you are still suffering ask him or her to refer you to a specialist pain or migraine clinic (see Appendix A).

Standard treatments for migraine

There are three standard ways to tackle migraine:

- Intervention to stop or minimise symptoms once a migraine has started.
  (The pharmaceutical approach is to constrict blood vessels directly by prescribing caffeine and/or ergotamine or by increasing serotonin levels.)
- Making yourself as comfortable as possible during a migraine
  (The pharmaceutical approach is to use pain-killers for the pain and anti-emetics for the nausea and vomiting.)
- Long-term treatment where the goal is to stop migraines occurring in the first place (by keeping blood vessels permanently open).

The ergotamine story

In the 19th century doctors and scientists noticed that the blood vessels leading to the brain tended to contract before a migraine and expand during an attack. They prescribed ergotamine which comes from ergot, a fungus that grows on rye. In the Middle Ages people who ate bread made with mouldy rye suffered a severe rash and their fingers and toes changed colour. In extreme cases their limbs developed gangrene and dropped off. The disease was known as 'St Anthony's fire' because sufferers went on pilgrimage to the shrine of St Anthony in Italy. During the months it took to get to the shrine they ate uncontaminated bread and their bodies 'miraculously' recovered from the ergot poisoning.

Ergotamine, like ergot, constricts blood vessels and is still in use today. Even if it doesn't cause gangrene it can make your hands and feet go white and cold. The main problem with it, however, is that when the effects of the ergotamine wear off blood vessels expand again and this can cause rebound headaches. These ergotamine-induced headaches can make you just as nauseous as migraine, but they tend to be dull, nagging and continuous. They can only be 'cured' by time or more ergotamine, so it's easy to get into an addictive spiral. The worse the rebound headache the larger the dose of ergotamine that's needed to 'cure' it, which makes the rebound headache even worse.

People suffering from ergotamine overdose may have to be taken into hospital when they are coming off the drug. Ergotamine is based on lysergic acid (part of the LSD family) and so can cause hallucinations. However ergotamine can be taken in moderation and it is a useful way to stop a migraine in an emergency – particularly if you get some warning and can take it at an early stage (see p 22). Although ergotamine has been used since the 19th century it doesn't work for everyone, and has obvious drawbacks. Modern drugs are thought to work in a similar way to ergotamine. They affect blood vessel contraction or dilation and serotonin.

How to use ergotamine

Common brand names: Cafergot, Wigraine, Medihaler
Ergotamine (aerosol), Ergomar, Ergostat (sublingual),
Bellergal, Bellergal-S

Ergotamine is not a pain-killer. It doesn't relieve pain
but encourages the blood vessels to remain constricted
and so stops the dilation of the blood vessels that causes
the headache and other symptoms that follow the aura.
If it doesn't work at the start of the migraine switch to
something else. If you are nauseous and vomit at the
very start of your migraine use a tablet that you can dissolve under your tongue (sublingual), or an inhaler or
suppository (inserted in the rectum). Ergotamine can be
useful if you don't get migraine very often – say, three or
four times a year – and can be helpful for cluster
headaches provided you stick to the recommended dose.
It's important to take ergotamine as early as possible –
ideally during the aura stage or when you get your first
warning of an approaching migraine.

People vary in their tolerance to ergotamine. The drug
stays in the body for a long time which is why periods of
rest from ergotamine are very important. Don't take
more than 6mg of ergotamine in any one week. Keep to
the lowest possible dose: half a tablet or half a suppository may be enough. Don't take more than four tablets
during one attack or more than six tablets in seven days.
Because it is so easy to become addicted ask your doctor
to monitor your usage carefully. Ask your doctor to
ration your prescriptions – or ask someone else to look
after your tablets.

Ergotamine is also available as:
● *Cafergot* – a mixture of ergotamine and caffeine that
  makes it work faster because caffeine also constricts
  blood vessels. A cup of coffee is cheaper if not as

convenient. Don't use if you hope to lie down and 'sleep off' the migraine.

- *Migril* – a mixture of ergotamine, caffeine and an anti-histamine. The caffeine makes it work faster but the anti-histamine may make you drowsy. Use if you have the chance to take things quietly and maybe sleep.

Short-term side-effects are nausea, rebound headache.* Long-term side-effects are gangrene of the limbs, addiction.

Other possible side-effects are blurred vision, drowsiness, dry mouth, palpitations, urinary retention, flushing, pins and needles*, diarrhoea, high blood pressure, leg cramps, abdominal pain, vertigo.

*Ask your doctor to help you stop taking the tablets if you are exceeding the stated dose or get pins and needles in your hands and feet. If you are taking ergotamine virtually every day and get daily headaches you may be suffering rebound headaches. Again, ask your doctor to help you cut down, and eventually stop taking the drug.

Do not take it if:

- you suffer from hyperthyroidism, heart, kidney, vascular or liver disease, high blood pressure, glaucoma or asthma
- you are elderly, pregnant or breast-feeding
- you are taking the painkiller 'Midrid', beta-blockers or the antibiotic *erythromycin*.

Modern drugs

In the 1970s a new drug *clonidine* (brand name Dixorit) began to be prescribed for migraine. Clonidine can cause tiredness, dizziness, dry mouth and dyspepsia. But despite the fact the original study was biased and later trials showed that it was no more effective than a

placebo (a dummy drug) it is still prescribed for
migraine as well as menopausal flushing.

Doctors accidentally discovered that the beta-blockers
they prescribed for high blood pressure and heart problems also help migraine. About a third of the people
who try the beta-blocker *propranolol*, for example, get
over 50 per cent fewer migraines. One of the best known
effects of beta-blockers is that they can make your hands
and feet cold and white, as contracting blood vessels
affects the circulation (see box on beta-blockers).
Calcium channel blockers have also been used to treat
migraine with similar success. They can cause night-
mares but this is rare if the dose is low enough.

Drugs for influencing serotonin levels – believed to be
a basic cause of migraine (see chapter 2, p. 17) – are *pizotifen* (brand name 'Sanomigran') and *sumatriptan* (brand
name 'Imigran').

Pizotifen, which reduces serotonin levels and needs to
be taken every day, stops the pre-migraine rise in serotonin. It is claimed to reduce the severity and frequency
of attacks in half of all sufferers. The commonest side-
effects are drowsiness, increased appetite and weight
gain. However it can also cause dizziness, dry mouth,
nausea and constipation. Sumatriptan is the latest drug
to act on serotonin levels. It boosts serotonin levels
which tells the blood vessels to contract. Sumatriptan is
sold as tablets or injections in the UK but it hasn't been
licensed in the US yet.

The advantage of sumatriptan is that it only affects
some of the brain's blood vessels, not all of them.
However, the most common side-effects are the result of
restricting the flow of blood to the brain: dizziness,
malaise and fatigue (see box opposite).

All about *sumatriptan* (UK brand name 'Imigran')

'I use Imigran for real emergencies. It's made it possible for me to be able to accept speaking engagements. Without reservation I can say yes, I will be there. Last week I had the start of a migraine when I woke up. I took half a tablet and was clear and able to be at the Migraine Doctor of the Year Award' – JO LIDDELL, DIRECTOR OF THE MIGRAINE ASSOCIATION (UK).

'I've been taking Imigran for two years. If I can take a tablet as soon as the headache begins it works. If it's too late to take a tablet I have an injection and I can literally feel it clear the migraine. I can feel it pushing up, going through my blood, clearing my headache. My husband says it even clears up my black eyes. I take it about once a week, at worst about three to four times a week. I try not to take it because I know it's expensive, so I'm conscious of not wasting them. At least I can take Imigran and I can function. I couldn't hold down a job before because I was sick too often' – SALLY, 41, LIBRARY ASSISTANT.

As Sally and Jo found out, sumatriptan can have a wonderfully liberating effect. It can be particularly helpful if you don't get migraines very often but are worried about making plans 'just in case' you get a migraine. But in spite of such glowing testimonials it is a drug, like all drugs, which must be used with care and has side-effects.

How to use it
Sumatriptan is available as tablets or injections. The tablets take 30 minutes to work, the injections 15 minutes. They are most useful if you get a warning aura and a gap before the full blown migraine starts. If you get little or no warning it's better to have the injections because the tablets won't get into your bloodstream by the time your migraine is in full swing.

Although the new auto-injectors are simple to use it is a good idea to ask your doctor or the nurse to show you how to do it and they will answer any of your questions. If it doesn't work first time don't try it again in the same attack.

Don't use it if:
- you are also taking other drugs, particulary ergotamine or anti-depressants
- you are very old, very young or pregnant
- you have high blood pressure or heart disease.

Side-effects of oral sumatriptan are malaise, fatigue, dizziness.

Side-effects of injected sumatriptan are pain where the needle goes in, tingling, heat, flushing, dizziness. It can also cause a sensation of heaviness, pressure, tightness, neck pain, drowsiness, weakness, increases in blood pressure, minor disturbances of liver function, vague discomfort in the chest, and it can also temporarily reduce the blood supply to the heart. There have also been reports of rapid and irregular heartbeats with palpitations and loss of consciousness. *Stop taking sumatriptan if you get chest pain or throat symptoms and tell your doctor about any adverse reactions.*

Points in favour of the drug
- It works for most people.
- It's selective.
- It enables you to make plans and to keep promises and commitments.

Points against
- It doesn't work for everyone.
- It's expensive.
- The long-term effects unknown.
- It's unsuitable for pregnant women.
- It's unsuitable for older people.
- It's unsuitable for children.
- Migraine may recur within 48 hours.

Sumatriptan compared with cafergot

In a controlled trial of 580 people sumatriptan was found to be more effective than the anti-migraine drug *cafergot* (ergotamine and caffeine) in relieving headache, nausea, light and sound sensitivity. However symptoms are more likely to return within 48 hours when taking sumatriptan than cafergot.

Continual use of cafergot can cause rebound headache so you mustn't take more than four in a 24-hour period and then you mustn't repeat the dose for another four days. Similar warnings are not given for sumatriptan – but this is a new drug and it took time for people to realize the rebound effect of ergotamine.

Other comparisons:

	Sumatriptan(%)	Cafergot (%)
Had another headache within 48 hours	41	30
Still nauseous after 2 hours	40	55
Still sensitive to light/sound after 2 hours	35	55
Improved after 2 hours	66	48

Long-term treatment

Conventional long-term (preventive) drug treatment takes time to work. It won't help with a migraine once it's started, and you need to check you can take normal treatments while the long-term ones are taking effect. For example, you can't take ergotamine with beta-blockers

Beta-blockers (drug names: *propranolol, nadolol, timolol*; brand names: Beta-Prograne, Betadur, Betaloc, Betim, Blocadren, Corgard, Inderal, Lopresor).

● 'With the beta-blockers I've put on a stone and a half in weight, but that's better than getting a migraine for three to five days every fortnight. I've been on beta-blockers for 12 years and tried to stop them. I keep a diary of my migraine and when I stopped taking the beta-blockers my diary went red with my marks for when I had migraine. Now I'm on new beta-blockers and you can see the difference in my diary' – Jo Liddell, director of the Migraine Association (UK).

● 'The drug stopped my symptoms. However I could not tolerate the drug's side-effects of breathlessness, fatigue, lethargy and insomnia' – Joan Sidwell.

Beta-blockers change the body's reaction to stress so it doesn't receive the normal messages to increase heart-rate and blood pressure. Not all beta-blockers are the same. If one beta-blocker doesn't work another one may. But beta-blockers are not suitable for people with asthma, diabetes, hypoglycaemia, low blood pressure, heart or chest problems. They can cause depression, sleep disturbances, insomnia, vivid dreams, fatigue, tiredness, lethargy, light-headedness, dizziness, nausea, gastro-intestinal upset, constipation, diarrhoea, bronchospasm, breathlessness, bradycardia, heart failure, cold extremities. They must not be used with the stomach-ulcer drug 'Tagamet' or ergotamine.

Calcium channel-blockers (drug names: *verapamil, nifedipine*; brand names: Berkatens, Cordilox, Geangin, Securon, Iniver, Isoptin, Procardia, Adalat, Coracten, Nifensar, Beta-Adalat, Tenif)

● 'I thought I was going to have a stroke on this drug. My head felt as if it were going to explode. The pressure was so intense I refused to continue using the drug. I could literally 'feel' the vasodilating properties of Isoptin. I later learned that the calcium channel-blockers are best taken when the cerebral arteries are in a state of rest, not after the headache has begun' – Betsy Wyckoff (*Overcoming Migraine*, Station Hill Press, USA, 1991).

Calcium channel-blockers make the blood vessels bigger and, though they are useful in the long-term treatment of migraine, should never be taken during a migraine: they will make it much worse. Common side-effects are headache, dizziness, flushing and oedema. Other side-effects are rash, constipation, nausea, vomiting, fatigue, light-headedness and increased urination. They should not be used if you are of childbearing age or have certain types of heart disease and sick sinus syndrome. They may cause problems if you have liver or kidney disease or if you are also taking beta-blockers or antihistamine. Calcium channel-blockers are not licensed for the treatment of migraine in the UK.

Other drugs your doctor may prescribe

- *Serotonin antagonists* (drug name: *methysergide*; brand name: Deseril): helpful for 27-57 per cent of people but because of side-effects treatment must be discontinued for at least one month in five. Adverse reactions include inflammation of the lining of the heart, lung and abdomen, arterial spasm, nausea, abdominal discomfort, tiredness, oedema, leg cramps, dizziness, drowsiness, weight gain, rash, hair-loss and central nervous system disturbances.
- *Alpha antagonists* (drug name: *clonidine*; brand name: Dixarit): no longer used much because the original trials on which it was granted a licence were found to be flawed. Nevertheless it has somehow retained its licence and is still in use. It is claimed to be useful for those sufferers whose attacks are associated with certain foods.
- *Anti-depressants*: migraine sufferers are more likely to be depressed than people who are not prone to migraine. But anti-depressants are prescribed for migraine because they affect serotonin production. If you are depressed the anti-depressants are less likely to help your migraine.

- *Non-steroidal anti-inflammatory drugs* (NSAIDs): mainly used for arthritis, these are sometimes prescribed because migraine is seen as a type of inflammation. They should always be taken with food to prevent nausea. But *don't take* NSAIDs if you have blood vessel disease, high blood pressure, kidney or liver disease, heart disease, glaucoma or asthma, or with the pain-killer 'Midrid' or beta-blockers. Side-effects include blurred vision, drowsiness, dry mouth, palpitations, urinary retention, flushing and pins and needles in the limbs. Tell your doctor if you get numbness or tingling.

Pain-killers and how to make the most of them

Pain-killers (also known as 'analgesics') contain one or more of the following:

- *Aspirin*: relieves pain and reduces inflammation and fever. Can damage the lining of the stomach, so avoid aspirin if you have a stomach ulcer.
- *Ibuprofen*: similar to aspirin, but less likely to cause stomach irritation. Not recommended if you have high blood pressure, kidney problems or stomach ulcer.
- *Paracetamol*: relieves pain and reduces fever. Not to be taken if you have kidney or liver problems.
- *Codeine*: related to morphine and only available in small quantities in non-prescription medicines. Found in combination with other pain-killing drugs. Even small doses can cause constipation.

Choosing the right cocktail

Some tablets contain caffeine which give you a bit of a lift – just what you need to get you home but a terrible idea if you want to rest and sleep. It's cheaper to take caffeine as a cup of coffee with your pain-killer than use pain-killers with added caffeine (but not so convenient if you're struggling to get home before your migraine develops). Some tablets contain anti-histamines that may help you to feel drowsy enough to rest.

Getting it down

Choose tablets that dissolve because they work quicker than non-soluble ones and are easier to swallow. You may find fizzy ones are easier to take if you are feeling nauseous. If you're out and about you might not have access to water and you may find that long thin tablets are easier to swallow than round ones.

Take tablets with warm water because they dissolve more easily. You may like to take it with sweet tea, but if there's milk in the tea it will take longer to digest. Pain-killers should be taken before meals so they are digested more quickly.

Getting the dose right

Read the instructions on the packet.

During a migraine attack you need between 600-900mg of aspirin for it to be effective. Each tablet of aspirin contains 300mg, so you need two to three. If the tablet also contains codeine it will have a stronger effect than aspirin alone.

Paracetamol comes in 500mg tablets and you need 1000mg, so take two tablets.

If you take too many pain-killers you can get withdrawal headaches. The more you take the more your body needs to feel normal. Withdrawal headaches can be a problem if you take over 1000mg of aspirin a day.

Paying too much?

There are huge variations in the cost of the different brands of pain-killers. Once you have found a pain-killer that works well for you ask your pharmacist if there are cheaper brands with the same ingredients.

Stronger pain-killers on prescription

Stronger pain-killers are available but only on prescription – that is, they must be authorized and sanctioned by a doctor. Your doctor may prescribe a mixture which will contain something for the nausea as well as something for the headache. For example, 'Paramex' (UK) is paracetamol and metaclopramide.

Do pain-killers work, and at what cost?

Americans use 20,000 tons of aspirin a year, or 225 tablets each at a cost of US$100 million. In the US at least half of headache patients are given no specific diagnosis, and are prescribed medication simply for pain relief. Less than 50 per cent of these report a reduction in symptoms with drug therapy and probably only a third receive sustained benefits. Increasing amounts of analgesics are used to obtain partial relief, leading to widespread abuse.

In Italy, they found that headache is the most frequent reason for the abuse of pain-killers and taking too many drugs (of any sort) is the biggest single reason why occasional headaches turn into chronic headaches.

Helping the medicine go down

Drugs can only work if they can reach your bloodstream, but one of the symptoms of migraine is that it slows your digestive processes to a standstill. Unless you take the drugs early in an attack you won't be able to digest the pain-killer in tablet form.

One way of coping with the nausea and vomiting is to take a pain-killer with *metoclopramide* which encourages gastric emptying – but this can cause diarrhoea. Other ways of overcoming the nausea and vomiting barrier is to get the medication into your system another way: take tablets that dissolve under the tongue and go straight into the bloodstream, inhale the medication or use suppositories.

Pain-killing drugs (analgesics)

'My doctor told me I had migraine and I asked him
how he knew. "Simple," he said, "you respond to
'Migraleve.' " – RICHARD BEALE.

Drug	Action	Side-effects
MIDRID	Analgesic	Dizziness
MIGRALEVE	analgesic, antihistamine	Drowsiness
MIGRAVESS	analgesic, anti-emetic	Drowsiness, diarrhoea, muscle-spasm, dizziness, insomnia, flatulence
MIGRIL	ergot /antihistamine/ xanthine cocktail	Rebound headache, abdominal pain, dry mouth, white cold hands and feet
PARAMAX	analgesic, anti-emetic	Drowsiness, diarrhoea
PERIACTIN	anti-histamine, serotonin antagonist	Drowsiness

Stop taking the tablets

It's so common for people to ditch the pills their doctors
prescribe that the doctors have their own name for this
phenomena: non-compliance. A UK survey found that
non-compliance can be as high as 92 per cent with short-
term drug regimes and an average of 50 per cent with
longer-term medications. The survey also found that of
the 30 per cent of migraine sufferers who see their doctor
only one in ten continue the recommended treatment.

If you are one of those, or even if you aren't, the gen-
tler aproaches outlined in the following chapters may be
more to your liking.

Should you go to a specialist migraine clinic?

'For the first time I felt my migraine was being taken seriously. The migraine clinic didn't dismiss it as just another headache' – FN.

The great advantage of going to a migraine clinic is, obviously, that they specialize in migraines. People who work there understand migraine in more depth than most family doctors. They will be able to tell you all about the latest treatments, offer you practical advice, and answer many of your questions. They may also ask you to take part in a trial. Some clinics (an example in Britain is the City of London Migraine Clinic) also offer help when you are in the middle of a migraine: a darkened room and a cup of tea.

You may not be able to find such a clinic in your area but many hospitals and medical schools now have their own pain clinics, where they also have a great deal of experience with migraine.

The Pain Evaluation and Treatment Institute of the University of Pittsburgh School of Medicine and a group of German researchers reviewed 65 pain studies and found that, on average, those of the 3,100 patients treated at specialist clinics showed a 56 per cent improvement in pain and disability compared with only 14 per cent improvement for people in the other groups.

You need to be referred by your doctor before you can go to some clinics.

CHAPTER 4

How to help yourself

Natural ways to avoid and stop migraine

The most impressive thing pharmaceutical drugs can do is stop a migraine in its tracks – but the 'natural way' can be equally impressive. Anybody who has had migraine knows that the migraine itself is 'natural'. This partially explains why so many people with migraine don't go to the doctor or take drugs for it. Many people instinctively realize that taking drugs to stop the migraine doesn't really solve anything, any more than disconnecting the temperature gauge of a car will stop it overheating. Taking drugs may make life more comfortable but doesn't get to the underlying cause of the problem.

Short-term self-help

> I get a pain under the arch of my feet or hands and a dull throbbing headache intermittently during the day, and then I know I'll wake up the next day at 6 am in blinding, agonizing pain' –
> MARK PAYNE.

We don't understand what causes migraine although we suspect that serotonin has something to do with it. One of the interesting things about serotonin is that it doesn't do anything directly – it just helps or hinders two nerve cells from communicating. Nerve cells join together to create different nerves in the body – and symptoms and cures depend on which nerve cells and nerves are affected. So treatment needs to be tailored to suit the individual.

Even the most effective drugs only work for some people – some of the time. But it's very little consolation to learn that a particular medicine helps 50 per cent of the people who try it if it doesn't help you. Treatment is largely a question of trial and error. There are no easy answers for migraine. Whatever you do it can take time and patience to find the treatment that works. The most important first step is to learn to recognize the warning signals (see chapter 2). If you tend to wake up with a migraine try and remember what happened to you the day before. If your migraine always catches you by surprise, get help. Ask your family, friends or colleagues at work. They might have noticed some tell-tale signs.

Provided you act quickly you can stop your migraine from developing, but you may have to experiment. Work methodically through the list below until you find a technique that suits you. Don't try everything at once.

1 Drink several glasses of water.
2 Drink sweet tea or coffee – caffeine to make your blood vessels contract, sugar for the energy boost (this may give only temporary relief).
3 Imagine your hands are warm or use other forms of relaxation imagery (see pp. 56, 107).
4 Lie down in a quiet, darkened room.
5 Do some exercise: for example, go for a run, jump up and down or make love. Sometimes stimulation will ward it off.
6 Go outside, especially if you're in a hot, stuffy room. Some people find that going out for a walk in the fresh air can ward off a migraine.
7 Have a hot bath or put your hands in warm water.
8 Massage your head, neck and shoulders (see box) – or press on the acupressure points (see figure 2).
9 Change your plans. If you have appointments cancel

Self-help massage

● Massage your feet or hands. This works in several ways: it relaxes tense muscles, warms up your feet or hands (which get cold as part of the body's natural response to stress) and diverts energy away from your head.

● Massage your neck and shoulders – to relax muscles that become increasingly tense before a migraine.

● Use your thumb or knuckle to apply pressure on the main 'headache' acupressure points: on your temples, on the back of your head, and the web of your hand between your thumb and forefinger. If you want more detailed help consult a recommended massage therapist (see chapter 10).

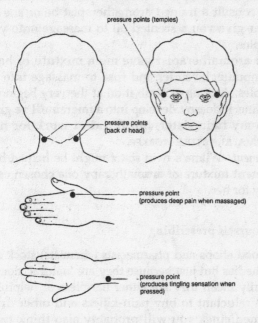

pressure points (temples)

pressure points (back of head)

pressure point (produces deep pain when massaged)

pressure point (produces tingling sensation when pressed)

Fig. 2 Pressure points

them. If you were going to spend time with your
family tell them you need time on your own – even if
your migraine doesn't develop.

10 Take the herb feverfew (see below 'Do-it-yourself
   prescribing').

11 Take vitamin B3 supplements (also known as 'niacin'
   or 'niacinamide'). The use of vitamin B3 has been
   used for counteracting the effects of LSD and it was
   discovered that some people find it helpful in stopping migraine. But beware: it dilates blood vessels
   and can make the migraine worse if taken in the middle of a migraine. Large doses are toxic and can also
   actually cause migraine.

12 Try aromatherapy, a massage with scented oils. If
   you consult a trained aromatherapist he or she can
   either give you a scented oil to massage onto your
   temples.
   'The aromatherapist gave me a mixture of basil,
   chamomile, lavender and rose to massage into my
   temples. As long as I rub it on at the very beginning
   I'm fine, it doesn't develop into a migraine. I've given
   it to my twin sister, but it didn't work for her.'
   – WILMA, 33, TEXTILE-WORKER.
   Comment Wilma's twin sister might be helped by a
   different mixture of aromatherapy oils chosen especially for her.

Do-it-yourself prescribing

Healthfood shops and pharmacists (chemists) stock natural remedies but just because they are 'natural' doesn't
necessarily mean they are either harmless or helpful. If
you are reluctant to buy pain-killers and other drug-
based medicines you will probably also think twice
about buying homoeopatic or herbal remedies or supple-
menting your diet with certain vitamins and minerals.

You may find that some of these remedies work for you – but they might not.

Buying a natural remedy on your own is largely a question of trial and error and if you are going to take a natural remedy it makes more sense to go to a professional practitioner who can prescribe something that is individually tailored to suit you. For example, *feverfew* is a common herb with anti-inflammatory properties thought to inhibit serotonin and is a well-known natural remedy for migraine if taken regularly over a period of time. However it doesn't suit everyone and it may be just one of a combination of herbs your body may need to get into balance.

Feverfew is a drug made from the dried leaves of a plant in the daisy family called *tanacetum parthenium* (figure 3) and can be bought at most healthfood stores and pharmacies. The herb is freeze-dried and sold in capsules. They can also be grown in the garden and eaten in a sandwich to disguise the slightly bitter taste. The recommended dose is 125mg a day but side-effects can be mouth-ulcers, itchy skin and sore throat. *Do not take* feverfew with drugs for high blood pressure or with alcohol.

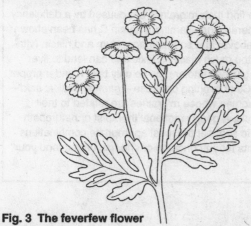

Fig. 3 The feverfew flower

'When I've felt a slight attack coming on, I take four feverfew tablets as often as I think I need to. I've taken as many as four lots of four in an afternoon and the attack has not come' – HOWARD HOPTROUGH.

'Feverfew didn't help me when I prescribed it for myself, but when I went to a medical herbalist it was one of the herbs he prescribed and my migraines started to get less frequent, and less severe' – JOAN CLARKE.

Some vitamins and minerals seem to help migraine, and some practitioners including medical doctors specialize in using them in mega-doses (*orthomolecular medicine* or *megavitamin therapy*). It worked for one man treated at the University of California Medical Center in San Francisco. His migraines disappeared (for the first time in six years) when he took 6gs of vitamin C but came back when his doctor gave him a placebo 'dummy' pill. Vitamin C helps the body fight disease and is one of the few vitamins the human body cannot produce for itself.

Vitamins and minerals helpful against migraine

Some people find their migraines are caused by a deficiency in certain minerals and vitamins. Vitamin C has been shown to help (see above) and so has magnesium and niacin (vitamin B3), but too much niacin is toxic and can lead to liver damage and glucose intolerance so only take it under proper supervision. Oil of evening primrose – *gamma linoleic acid* – has helped women whose migraines are related to their menstrual cycle. A good nutritional therapist or naturopath may be able to suggest the most appropriate combinations of supplements for you once he or she has understood your case fully.

Long-term self-help strategy

If you suffer from migraine you may feel that what you're really suffering from is an overload – your body is trying to balance you in the best way it knows how, by forcing you to retreat. Could this be why migraine gives you every encouragement to lie down in a quiet darkened room? Is it your body's way of saying no?

This doesn't mean that migraine is your fault – any more than it's someone's fault if they have a natural tendency towards ulcers, heart problems or asthma. We all have different tendencies, different ways in which we react to the stresses and strains of life. For example, under stress some people will always tend to put on a lot of weight whereas others will lose weight, some will get psoriasis, others will lose the pigment in their skin. In the same way some people suffer from headaches and others suffer from migraine – and some people sometimes have headaches and sometimes have a migraine. Everyone reacts to the inner and outer stresses of life in their own way. No-one is protected. 'Your way' may be to have migraine. If so, what are the 'natural' ways you can help yourself?

If you want to change something it is important to start with some idea of where you are in the first place. Just as migraine may have more than one cause it may need more than one approach to deal with it. So it will help to take a good long look at yourself from the mental, physical and emotional perspective. Keeping a diary can be an important first step that will help you in all sorts of different ways. At the very least put a big red cross on the calendar every time you have a migraine (and if you're a woman you should also mark down when you have your period).

Making sense of your migraine

Something as simple as keeping a 'migraine diary' can tell you a lot about the *pattern* of your migraine. You may be more likely to get one just before your period, or just before your bank statement arrives, or on Saturday mornings. Identifying the pattern of your migraine is an important part of helping yourself (see box 'Common triggers for migraine').

It will prove useful as you try different treatments. After all, if you don't know how often you have migraine before you start treatment, how will you know what difference the treatment itself has made?

Also, if you decide to see a natural health practitioner they might ask questions about what makes your migraine better or worse, or whether you've noticed if your migraines follow particular patterns. Keeping a diary will make these sort of questions easier to answer.

The diary should be easy to use and give you a clear picture of what you are doing and eating before a migraine starts. It shouldn't be so detailed that you have to wade through masses of paper to get to the important information. The sort of things to write down are:

- The foods you suspect of contributing to your migraine. You might also find it useful to note down anything you've eaten that's particularly unusual.
- Anything else you feel may be contributing to your migraine such as shopping, travelling, watching television, working with a computer and so on.

On migraine days write down:
- When it started.
- When it finished.
- Major symptoms (aura, vomiting, nausea, headache and so on).
- The effect of any medication or self-help treatment:

Common 'triggers' for migraine: Check-list

- not enough food (see page 49):
    - skipping meals (whatever happened to lunch?)
    - skimping meals (a slice of toast isn't enough)
- migraine foods (see page 46):
    - chocolate
    - cheese
    - red wine
    - any alcohol
    - coffee
    - any caffeine (some migraine tablets contain caffeine).
    See fuller list in box 'Suspect foods', p. 46.
- women's hormones
    - menstruation
    - pregnancy
    - hormone replacement therapy (HRT)
    - contraceptive pill
    - menopause
- sleep
    - too much (lying-in)
    - too little (over-tired)
- 'mechanical' problems (see chapter 8):
    - jaw (teeth-grinding, teeth-clenching, temporal mandible dysfunction)
    - neck (tension, posture, whiplash injury)
    - back
    - sinuses
    - eyes (eye-strain)
    - teeth
- environment:
    - bright flickering lights
    - exercise
    - shopping
    - travelling
    - weather
    - strong smells
    - VDUs
- emotions (see chapter 9):
    - stress at home or work
    - depression

did the pain-killer work, did a warm bath help?

- What you think might have brought it on: food, wine, pressure at work, missed meals, exercise. Is there any emotional stress that you think could be connected to the migraine?

On non-migraine days write down what you did and ate and how you feel.

The food factors

'I didn't recognize it as migraine at first. I was in my twenties, getting married, having children, changing jobs, studying for professional exams, changing houses. I suppose it was quite a stressful time. It happened every three months or so. I saw stars, then I had a violent headache that was always on the right side of my temple and round the back of my head. I didn't actually vomit but I felt nauseous. I had to sit down or lie down. In those days one didn't think of migraine as an illness, it was just something that attacked for some unknown reason.

'There was a time when I didn't get them very often and then they started to get much worse. I got them about once a week and they were very painful. I have never suffered such violent headaches before or since. I had started to get interested in alternative health and I read somewhere that migraine could be caused by dairy products, chocolate and stress. I remember pinpointing an attack to just after I'd had an iced chocolate cake with chocolate cream in the middle. I thought, well, I might just as well try it. I came off chocolate and dairy products and the migraines disappeared just like that. It was remarkable.

'That was in 1981 and I've only had two minor attacks since. I stick to the diet fairly rigidly. I used to adore chocolate, now I just eat carob and I steer clear of cream and other dairy products. I regret not being able to eat these things but it doesn't really bother me, although I may have a bit of cheese or take milk in my tea when I visit friends.

'I also have feverfew handy. When I've felt a slight attack coming on I take four tablets. I've taken as many as four lots of four in an afternoon and the attack has not come. I get a little whirring, slight nausea and perhaps a twinge in the head. I've not tried it without the feverfew. Knowing what I do about the attacks I do everything I can to stop them'
— HOWARD HOPTROUGH, 70, RETIRED COLLEGE LECTURER.

Like Howard, you may find that eating certain foods like chocolate will always bring on a migraine, but a little bit of milk doesn't do any harm. Or you may find that you can sometimes get away with certain foods if you are not overloaded with other stresses. For example, some women can eat chocolate and cheese quite happily three weeks out of four but find these foods will always give them a migraine in the week before their period.

We know that rain comes from clouds but it doesn't always rain when its cloudy. Although we can't predict the weather you may be able to anticipate the times when certain foods are most likely to bring on your migraine. For example, you may be able to eat a chocolate, but a bar of chocolate instead of lunch is asking for trouble. It's the combination that tips the balance between what you can cope with and what you can't. Also, it's the times when you are tired or stressed or pre-menstrual that you're most likely to forget that certain foods may bring on a migraine.

Suspect foods

- any food that increases serotonin levels is suspect. For example, foods with an 'amine' in it, such as cheese (tyramine), chocolate (phenylethyl*amine*) and citrus fruit (octop*amine*).
- foods with the amino acid *tryptophan*, such as milk or turkey.

Other key suspects:

- *monosodium glutamate* (also known as MSG), a food additive found in instant rice, soup, TV dinners, instant gravy, potato chips, meat tenderizers and seasoning. The MSG in Chinese food is so famous for provoking migraines that it's known as the 'Chinese Restaurant Syndrome'.
- nitrates – found in smoked and processed meats such as hot dogs, bacon, ham, salami, sausage, pepperoni
- caffeine – found in coffee, tea and fizzy cola drinks
- chicken livers

Miscellaneous suspects:

- fruit and vegetables such as bananas, canned figs, dates, raisins, strawberries, avocados, papaya, pineapples, red plums, raspberries, mangoes, spinach, various beans (soybeans, lima beans, pinto beans etc), onions, olives, eggplant (aubergines), Italian broad beans, pea-pods, sauerkraut, lentils, snow peas (mange tout), pickles, tomatoes, nuts and peanut butter, potatoes, sunflower seeds, pumpkin seeds, sesame seeds, soy products (bean curd, miso soup), garlic
- meat and fish such as liver, sweetbreads, kidneys, brains, gamemeats, salted or smoked fish (smoked salmon, anchovies), pickled herring, pork, preserved meat, caviare, chicken livers, pâté
- dairy products such as cream, yoghurt, cheese (except cream cheese and cottage cheese), sour cream, buttermilk, eggs
- cereal products such as corn, wheat
- alcoholic drinks such as beer, sherry, red wine

- seasonings such as vinegar
- fungus such as yeast
- sweets such as liqorice, the sugar substitute 'aspartame'

Foods with no known headache-causing potential
- Lamb, chicken, pears, unsweetened pear juice, brussel sprouts, zucchini, cauliflower, carrots, broccoli.

If your migraines are brought on by certain foods you may be suffering from a 'food sensitivity' or 'food intolerance'. Keeping a diary will help you to identify the foods you are sensitive to. If you suspect a certain food, leave it out of your diet for several weeks and see if it affects your migraine. Only eliminate one food at a time. If you always get a migraine when you eat even a small amount of certain foods you may have an intolerance to them. People who have intolerances to certain foods and chemicals are usually thought of as having an 'allergic reaction' to those foods (or, at least, the chemicals in them). Migraine can be just such a reaction – although it is not, strictly medically-speaking, an allergy. If you think your migraine is caused by a food sensitivity or intolerance see a specialist.

Diagnosing food intolerances

Many natural therapists specialize in discovering and treating food sensitivities, especially those using 'applied kinesiology' (also known as 'Touch for Health') and 'clinical ecology'.

Applied kinesiologists use muscle-testing to help you discover the foods most likely to give you migraine. This is based on the idea that if a food affects you it can also affect certain muscles. In other words, it doesn't just give you migraine it makes all your muscles weaker. The therapist applies pressure to your arm to test your strength when there is nothing in your mouth, and re-tests when you have a sample of the suspect food under your tongue. There is, however, no independent evidence that the test is accurate.

Clinical ecologists may give you drops of suspect foods or, less common now, they may inject your skin with them. If you are sensitive to the food your skin quickly becomes inflamed. Such therapists are often medical doctors (by law injections can only usually be carried out by medically-qualified people in most countries). They may also help you by monitoring you during an elimination diet where what you eat is severely restricted to non-headache causing food and then suspect foods are re-introduced one food at a time.

Once you've found the foods that cause migraine, what then? There are various options. You can:

● build yourself up to such an extent that you are no longer sensitive to these suspect foods.

● eliminate these foods altogether – which means constantly watching what you eat and drink.

● be de-sensitized to your culprit foods by taking drops that are samples of food diluted to the correct 'homoeopatic strength'. This shouldn't be confused with classical homoeopathy where a single homoeopatic remedy is chosen to match the individual (not the individual's sensitivity).

Migraine and diet

There are a million interesting theories about diet but few clear answers. The only real question is what kind of diet do you feel healthiest on? The choice is almost endless: the raw food diet, the macrobiotic diet, food combining or Hay diet, the Wright diet, the Pritkin diet, the Plus-Minus diet, and so it goes on. All we really know is that some diets work for some people but not for others.

The Hay diet

Although this diet is designed for people who suffer from digestive problems some people have found that their migraines disappear when they go on it. It was devised by the American doctor William Howard Hay (1866-1940) who believed that protein stimulates the production of acid in the stomach, which interferes with the digestion of carbohydrates. Hay recommended that you don't eat carbo-hydrates and proteins (or fruit which is an acid food) in the same meal. It may work for people who are prone to migraine simply because the digestive system isn't over-loaded.

Other Hay rules are:
- cut down on proteins, starches and fats
- cut down on refined foods such as white flour and sugar.

If your migraines coincide with sugar 'lows' or if you wake up with them make a conscious effort to eat 'prop-erly' every four hours. That means don't skip or skimp on meals, have a warm milky drink at bedtime, and you might even find it helps to have a sandwich as well. This is a very common suggestion, but it's also slightly odd. Warm milk contains tryptophan, which is converted into serotonin. Serotonin levels rise before a migraine, and it's one of the foods that some people have to avoid. This is but one of many examples where the very thing that helps some people with migraine actually causes migraine in others.

If you tend to suffer from migraine when you are on a sugar 'low' – when the level of sugar in your blood is low – your insulin production may be the culprit. In some people, refined sugar stimulates the pancreas to release excess insulin that metabolizes not only the sugar just eaten but also any sugar already present in the bloodstream. The result is a lower blood sugar level than before. If you avoid sugar you avoid this particular rollercoaster. If you are going to kick the sugar habit you need to eat plenty of brown rice, wholemeal bread and pasta (or any other *unrefined* carbohydrate) with every meal. High protein snacks (cheese, meat, fish, peanut butter and so on) are best.

Tackling the obvious things first

Certain things create headaches for most people – but they only bring on a migraine if you have a tendency towards migraine. They are:

Alcohol

People vary in their tolerance to alcohol. Most people who suffer from migraine can't drink red wine. If you are serious about tackling your migraine give up alcohol altogether and see if this helps. If you can't cut down your consumption consult a therapist who can help you (see chapter 9).

Drugs

Many drugs can contribute to migraine. Any drug with the word 'amine' in the name is a potential suspect (for example, ergotamine: see chapter 3) but other drugs can also contribute to your migraine. Consult your doctor. Ask him or her if you can stop taking the tablets. Does this make any difference to your migraine? Non-prescription drugs, cigarettes and even caffeine can cause migraine. Do you depend on these or other 'recreational chemicals' and stimulants? Can you stop using them and see whether it gets rid of your migraine? If you can't then consult a therapist who can help you (see chapter 9).

Vitamin pills

Large doses of vitamin B can cause migraine. So can large doses of vitamin E. Some vitamin tablets contain soy yeast and other food products that may bring on a migraine. Stop taking the pills and see what happens.

Foods

Chocolate, cheese, coffee, peanuts, oranges (and other citrus fruits) are common migraine triggers. You can experiment by avoiding these foods (see food box on page 46).

Physical risk factors

Have a thorough physical check-up and also consider factors in your daily surroundings that might be to blame. For example, your posture, or even the chair you sit in may be contributing to your migraine (see chapter p. 99).

Psychological risk factors

Talk over your mental and emotional state with a good therapist (see chapter 9). People who suffer from migraine are more likely to be depressed – simply because of the pain. If you are depressed you are more likely to feel isolated, have trouble sleeping (or wake up early), and you may lose your appetite for food and/or sex.

Learning how to dodge the main triggers

Identifying and controlling the factors that bring on your migraine helps some people some of the time. In one study attack frequency was reduced by nearly half in a group of people who identified and learned to control their risk factors.

If you notice that you often get a migraine after eating chocolate steer clear of chocolate. If you notice that you often get a migraine when you drink wine steer clear of wine. This may be easier said than done. If you get a migraine ten minutes after eating chocolate the chocolate may be the culprit – or it may be that the craving for chocolate is an indication you are about to have a migraine.

You can also try to avoid situations that seem to bring on your migraine. For example, if you have Saturday morning migraines try getting up at your normal work-day hour. Some so-called migraines are caffeine withdrawal headaches. People who drink lots of coffee at work during the week get withdrawal symptoms on Saturday mornings. You can get over this problem by weaning yourself off coffee altogether (do it gradually, otherwise you'll get an awful withdrawal headache) – or you can make your addiction part of your lifestyle and be sure that you have a cup of coffee with your Saturday morning lie in.

You may find that your migraines happen when you've missed a meal, or if there is a long time between meals. Make a conscious effort to eat a 'proper' (that is, cooked) meal every four hours.

You may find that it's fairly easy to prevent a migraine by some simple changes in eating habits or lifestyle. On the other hand, you may find that it's either quite difficult for you to change or your migraine may be brought on by situations you simply can't avoid – such as shopping. You may need to seek professional support to help you change what you do (such as skip-ping meals) or your reactions to the inevitable and unavoidable (such as shopping). You may also find that you are more likely to suffer from a migraine if you are under stress and you may want to take a closer look at how you handle stress – and relaxation. We'll deal with this next.

CHAPTER 5

Activating your own
healing system

*How relaxation, biofeedback and
meditation can help*

'I don't remember a time when I didn't get them. I
felt sick in my stomach and dizzy and my vision
went funny. It usually happened before something
exciting like a circus, a party, that sort of thing.
When I got older I got them because of achieve-
ment-orientated stress. I needed to do really, really
well. It was a "be perfect" thing for me. It wasn't
good enough to get Bs in class, it had to be As. Low
blood sugar might also have been a trigger because I
tend not to eat when I'm under stress.

'The first thing I felt was a distance, as if I was
wandering along two feet behind and above my
head. The next symptom was usually being sick in
my stomach, vomiting, and feeling cold and shaky
and still having that feeling of everything happening at a distance. The lights hurt my eyes and I
wanted to hide under the bed. I had difficulty
speaking, my tongue got wrapped round my eye
teeth and I couldn't see what I was saying.
Something happens that disconnects your brain
from your ears, your eyes and your mouth and if
you're really unlucky, from your hands and feet.

'I only realized it was migraine when I was in my
late thirties or early forties, when I went to college

and the instructor described classic migraine. I started using the biofeedback technique she'd been talking about to help my migraine – and it worked. As soon as I started getting that spaced-out feeling I used the biofeedback idea, but without the instruments. I visualized my hands getting warmer and imagined holding my hands in hot water and relaxing until my hands warmed back up.

'If I remembered to do that before I got sick it would go. Then, after a while, I stopped having them. I was meditating more and handling stress better. I also started to change my attitude and tried to stop expecting too much of myself. Now, when I catch myself trying to be perfect or criticizing myself for not achieving perfection, I stop and say I don't have to do this, and I have a little laugh at myself. I try to be gentle and understanding with myself.

'I haven't had a migraine in years, but if I let my blood sugar get too low, lights bother me, my hands go cold, I have verbal dyslexia and I just want to crawl away somewhere. But it's only low blood sugar and it goes away as soon as I eat something.'
– JESSICA MACBETH, HEALER.

The American healer Jessica Macbeth, who describes her own battle against migraine above, learned how to control her migraines by relaxing, meditating and changing her attitude to life. Her book *Moon Over Water* (see Appendix B) is recommended reading for anyone with migraine who wants to learn how to meditate to counteract migraine naturally.

Relaxation

The physiological effects of relaxation include the following:

- lower heart rate and blood pressure
- lower respiratory (breathing) rate
- lower blood lactic acid levels
- lower oxygen consumption
- lower muscle tension
- lower adrenalin levels
- lower blood cortisone levels
- increase in the flow of nutrients through the body's internal organs
- increase in skin temperature
- increase in electrical resistance of skin

If we change any one of these physical symptoms it also changes the rest. Just increasing skin temperature can have a ripple effect. If you are feeling stressed and your hands are cold it can be relaxing simply to warm your hands and feet. But stress patterns are also interlinked. For example, if your breathing is stuck in your upper chest, in an alarm pattern, it will force the rest of your body to stay in stress. As an experiment try sitting with your shoulders deliberately tensed-up and your jaw clenched. Note how you feel. That's what you have to try to change.

Learning to relax takes time and practice, particularly if you have spent most of your life being tense. So don't underestimate the challenge nor the amount of support and teaching you might have to find. You might find it helpful to read other books, go to relaxation classes, use tapes or ask friends what they do. If you want to be able to ward off a migraine before it starts you need to practise relaxation until it's easy and automatic. Practise every day – if necessary, twice a day. You may find that learning to relax has a spin-off effect and the migraines themselves will become less frequent and less severe.

There are several different methods of relaxation you might find useful:

- Gently tightening and then letting go of the tension in groups of muscles in turn, working your way up from your toes to your head.
- Telling yourself that groups of muscles are warm and heavy, or warm and soft, again working your way up from your toes to your head. Avoid the word 'relaxation'. There's nothing quite like being told to relax to make you want to tense up.
- You can also imagine yourself in pleasant, relaxing surroundings – in a beautiful garden or on a warm beach for example (this technique is known as 'imagery').
- There are many relaxation tapes on the market (audio and video) and you may find it helpful to play one of these. The British Holistic Medical Association, for example, produce them as part of its Tapes for Health series (see Appendix A). The only way to find out if a particular tape is relaxing is to try it. You'll know if it works if you feel calmer and more peaceful afterwards.

More relaxation methods

Doing anything that makes you feel relaxed can be helpful in averting a migraine – or make having one less likely:

- Relaxing in a warm bath or under a warm shower increases skin temperature and may make muscles less tense. The most complete version of this is floating in a flotation tank – possibly the most relaxing experience in

Bank managers or tigers: Fighting the 'fight or flight' response

The primitive part of our brain doesn't understand the difference between an angry boss or bank manager and a charging sabre-toothed tiger. Faced with any kind of danger the brain signals alarm, which the body responds to by producing stress hormones such as adrenalin to handle the emergency. The body is ready to fight or run away – the famous 'fight or flight' response. Muscles tighten up ready to run, the heart starts to pound, we breathe more rapidly and our feelings may range from simple unease to overwhelming panic. As blood is diverted to our essential organs, our fingers and toes may even start to look white and feel cold as they receive less blood. Long-term, lower level worries have the same effect on us.

If we survived the danger of the sabre-toothed tiger we could relax. The fight or flight response would have worn itself out and we would be left with the symptoms of relaxation. These 'symptoms' include a feeling of warmth and heaviness, slow even breathing, steady heart rate and a sense of well-being and relief. Unfortunately, bank managers and modern sources of stress don't help us to exercise away our stress hormones as efficiently as sabre-toothed tigers and although we produce the same physical reactions to stress, we've nowhere to run to and nothing to fight. We're left with all the stress symptoms of tight muscles, pounding heart, rapid breathing and feelings of panic. When the stress is over it's sometimes difficult to persuade ourselves that the danger is over and it's time to relax. We get stuck in a stress pattern.

When we are ready for danger, or relaxing after stress, our hormones affect us in ways that encompass body, mind and emotion – and these are all interdependent. It's impossible to feel physically relaxed if we are mentally or emotionally stressed. How we think affects how we feel physically and emotionally. How we feel physically affects how we feel emotionally and how we think.

the world. In a flotation tank, which is an enclosed chamber, you float effortlessly in skin-temperature water saturated with Epsom salts. Some people feel as refreshed after an hour's float as if they've had a fortnight's holiday. Some flotation tanks are totally silent, others have underwater speakers that can be used to provide soothing music or hypnosis tapes.

- Massage is relaxing because it helps to release tension from the muscles.
- Some people find that exercise is relaxing – perhaps because it gives the 'fight or flight' stress hormones something useful to do and uses them (see box on page 57).

But a word of warning: If you finally relax after years of being tense you may feel very tired. This doesn't mean that the relaxation made you tired – it just means that for the first time in a long time you are noticing how your body really feels. The relaxation has simply put you in touch with the stress and exhaustion your body may have been experiencing for some time. Once you've caught up with yourself and had the rest you need relaxation exercises will enable you to feel refreshed.

Biofeedback

Biofeedback relies on the fact that the body responds to stress and relaxation in ways that can be measured by machines (figure 4). For example, relaxation results in a rise in skin temperature whereas stress makes your skin colder as blood is diverted to the lungs, heart and other muscles that are essential for the 'flight or fight' mechanism.

The most common way of using biofeedback for migraine is to imagine that your hands are warm and then your skin temperature is 'fed back' to you. If your

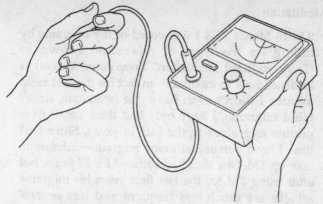

Fig. 4 A basic biofeedback machine

hands are warm you're relaxed, and if they're cold you're stressed. The 'feedback' is usually a machine that measures finger-tip temperature in tenths of a degree. You can also use an ordinary room thermometer that only changes when you've warmed up by a whole degree.

The Neurologic Center for Headache and Pain in La Jolla, California, has had considerable success with biofeedback. Over an average of 14 sessions people have reduced the frequency and severity of their migraines by 87 per cent. Research in the US, Holland and Sweden has shown that biofeedback helps between 40 and 60 per cent of people with headaches.

Seeing or hearing a change in the biofeedback machine can help you relax because it reassures you that your skin temperature is really changing. But you shouldn't become hooked on using the machine. As Jessica Macbeth found out you don't need biofeedbac' machines to relax. US research has shown that relaxati' training alone produced a 38 per cent improvemen' migraine sufferers.

Meditation

'On 16 March 1974 I was cured of my migraine by taking up the form of relaxation known as 'Transcendental Meditation'. I was cured as soon as I learned how to meditate – in fact for the first eight months I didn't even have one headache, never mind migraine. I have only had three small five-minute migraines in the last 19 years. Since that time I have persuaded many migraine-sufferers to take up TM. One man had suffered for 27 years, but after using TM for the last four years his migraine attacks are much less frequent and less severe'
– A F.

'The week after I learned TM I suffered a slight migraine which lasted for two days – very different to the severe migraines I had been having. From then on for the whole of 1990 and into 1991 I did not have a migraine, despite taking on extra workloads during that time' – A E D.

Transcendental Meditation, better known just as 'TM', is the brand name for the kind of meditation the Beatles learned in the 'swinging 60s' from the Maharishi Mahesh Yogi. Today it is practised by about four million people all over the world. The technique is to repeat a single word (*mantra*) for 15-20 minutes twice a day.

However not everybody eliminates their migraines by learning TM in particular or meditation in general. In the UK about 600 doctors practise TM – but some of them still get migraine, as the following examples illustrate:

'I've tried everything, all the usual pain-killers, I even resorted to *pethidine* (Demerol) when the pain was unbearable. I've tried yoga, meditation, acupuncture, homoeopathy, everything. The only relief I get is on holiday – but it comes back when I go back to work' – DR H.

'Meditation has not affected the pattern of my migraine but it may have stopped them being really bad every time. I've been meditating regularly for at least 12 years, and started yoga 18 years ago but I don't think it's really helped' – J N.

Meditation is unlikely to help your migraines if you are not physically relaxed. Some people meditate in ways that reduce mental stress, but not physical stress. Silently repeating a mantra may be very calming and cure some people of migraine, but it will only work if they manage to become relaxed physically as well as mentally. If your hands are cold after 20 minutes meditating your body is still not relaxed and you may need to change your method of meditation.

Breathing holds the key. If you breathe mostly with your upper chest this is the type of breathing associated with stress. It's impossible to relax if you are breathing as if you are running away from danger. Similarly, it's hard to feel tense if your breathing is slow and deep – as if you were sleeping soundly. Don't confuse deep breathing with taking big breaths. Some people think that deep breathing means pulling in their stomach and breathing from the upper chest. It's not. If your stomach doesn't move when you are breathing you're not breathing deeply. And if you're not breathing deeply – from your stomach – you're not breathing properly, or well.

If your body has been in a tense state for a long time it may take several years to reduce your body's underlying habit of alarm, so it's important to concentrate on physical relaxation first.

Learning simple meditation

Meditation is a simple way to learn how to relax your body as well as your mind and one of the easiest ways is focusing on the breath. Just by observing your natural breath can relax you quickly and easily. For example, in *Moon Over Water* Jessica Macbeth describes an exercise in which you stare at your thumbnail and count your breath. Keeping your eyes open and focused during this meditation is particularly helpful if you are the sort of person who can feel wonderfully calm and peaceful while they meditate but start to tense up again as soon as they open their eyes.

When you relax, your brainwave frequencies are mainly in slow cycle *alpha* waves. When you meditate they go into *alpha* and *theta*, an even more deeply relaxed and stable state.

Relaxation and stress

Unpublished UK research by a physiotherapist-turned-acupuncturist at the York Headache Clinic has found that both relaxation and acupuncture help migraine with a 59 per cent reduction in headache-hours. The interesting thing about this research is that during both treatments people were encouraged to take responsibility for their own situation and not to rely on drugs. As they started to develop control, choice and skill in dealing with the source of the stresses in their lives they made significant changes in their lifestyles – changing jobs, moving house and so on. While they were in the process of making these changes they were creating stressful situations. In the short-term this *increased* their stress levels, but because they were dealing with the underlying issues they *reduced* their headaches.

Does your sensitivity give you migraine?

If you are sensitive enough to be disturbed by computer screens and flickering lights, you may also experience involuntary psychic sensitivity. You may feel overwhelmed by the energy of crowds, and don't like shopping or pubs because there are so many people there and you are likely to pick up lots of garbled psychic energy. It is as if you have a television which picks up all the TV stations at once.

Many people who get migraine have a reticular activating system (RAS) that doesn't filter out much information (see page 14 'All about the brain') and this may be the cause. The best way to 'turn down' your RAS is to practise meditation. However it takes time to re-train your nervous system so be patient. If you want a temporary filter try tinted glasses, particularly if your migraine often starts when you've been reading or in bright sunlight. Recent research has shown that people with migraines often come from families with dyslexia – and that both are helped by tinted glasses. People with migraine often find blue or green-tinted glasses helpful, but steer clear of rose-tinted spectacles (seriously!).

CHAPTER 6

The natural therapies and migraine

Introducing the 'gentle alternatives'

Doctors and natural therapists come in many different hues. Some are 'gardeners' and others are 'mechanics'. Mechanics want to fix people like they are fixing a machine. They see people's diseased 'parts' and want to change them or replace them. Some doctors and natural therapists treat only the symptoms, the outward signs of the disease, and always give people with migraine the same pill, potion or treatment.

Gardeners, on the other hand, do whatever they can to support you and help you grow. The doctor who suggested that someone with migraine join the British Migraine Association was a 'gardener' – that is, giving someone support and useful advice to help them grow and heal themselves. Doctors who suggest you keep a migraine diary are also gardeners. These are people who realize that you are more than a collection of symptoms and that your mind also needs to be involved in the process of getting well. For obvious reasons therapies that concentrate on this relationship between mind and body are sometimes called body-mind therapies.

Some doctors and therapists go further and treat the individual as a combination of mind, body, emotions and spirit. This is known as the 'holistic' approach since it treats people as a natural 'whole'. It is for this reason that those therapies that aim to treat 'the whole person' are sometimes known as 'whole person therapies' or 'whole system therapies'.

Different people have different ideas about what is holistic and natural and what isn't. But here are some ideas common to most natural therapies, which might help you to recognize the 'mechanics' from the 'gardeners'.

The principles of natural therapy

- The human being is a subtle and complex blend of body, mind, emotions, and spirit – all of which are interconnected and any one of which may cause or contribute to health or disease.
- The body has a natural ability to heal itself. Whereas some doctors and scientists dismiss the so-called 'placebo effect' as 'only the body healing itself' natural therapies are about encouraging the body to do just that.
- Good health is a state of mental, emotional and physical 'balance.' Symptoms may provide a way for an individual who moves away from this ideal balance to cope with internal and external stress – in other words, a symptom is a way of *getting back* to balance (for example, if you need to rest you have a migraine which forces you to rest).
- Environmental and social conditions are important to a person's physical and psychological well-being and may have an important impact on their health.
- Treating the root cause or causes of a problem – that is, what makes someone susceptible to a problem such as migraine and what triggers it off – is more important than treating the obvious immediate symptoms. Treating only symptoms may simply cover up the underlying problem and make it worse, so that it reappears later as something much more serious (see also the 'Law of Cure', page 79).

- Each individual is unique and cannot be treated in exactly the same way as any other individual.
- Healing is usually quicker and more effective if the person takes responsibility for their own health and, wherever and whenever possible, has an active involvement in the healing process.
- There is a natural healing 'force' or 'energy' in the universe. The Chinese call this *qi* or *chi* (pronounced 'chee'), the Indians *prana*, and western healers variously *vis medicatrix naturae*, 'spirit' and 'life force'. We use this energy to maintain well-being and heal ourselves, and we use this same energy when we are ill. Some therapists work directly with this energy, strengthening and balancing their client's life-force, so helping them to heal themselves.
- Natural therapies are based on the principles of the healers of ancient Greece and Egypt: to cause no harm, to treat the individual as a whole, and to encourage people to take an active part in their own recovery and health maintenance.
- Good natural therapists are aware that in order to help heal their clients they must know themselves and be actively engaged in healing themselves.

How natural therapies treat migraine

Some natural therapies act directly on the migraine in a purely physical way much like a drug (for example, the herbal remedy feverfew does this). Others work on the underlying causes and try to get to the root of the problem. Psychological therapies try to get to the cause of the problem by working with the mind and emotions, the physical therapies (such as osteopathy) work with the body and the energy therapies (such as acupuncture) work with the 'energy' body.

Natural therapies effective in treating migraine

The following is a list of the therapies effective in treating your migraine safely, effectively and above all gently – without drugs:

Proven
- Acupuncture
- Biofeedback
- Chiropractic
- Healing (faith/spiritual healing)
- Herbalism
- Homoeopathy
- Hypnosis/hypnotherapy
- Yoga.

Other approaches that may be useful
- Acupressure (including Shiatsu)
- Aromatherapy
- Bioenergetics
- Colour therapy
- Crystal therapy
- Dance therapy
- Massage
- Meditation
- Naturopathy
- Osteopathy
- Physiotherapy/Physical therapy
- Polarity therapy
- Psychotherapy/Counselling
- Radionics
- Reflexology
- Rolfing
- Traditional Chinese medicine
- Vacuflex therapy
- Visualization.

Choosing a natural therapy

It's very important to try one therapy at a time – and give that therapy time to work. How can you tell which therapy is working if you're trying half a dozen at the same time? Don't become a therapy-junkie. Stick with one therapy until you know whether it works or not. Don't confuse the issue by trying everything at once.

In some ways it doesn't really matter which therapy you choose. Just to be attracted to a particular therapy may mean it is the right one for you. Many people have an intuitive feeling about which therapy is most likely to help them.

Points to remember in getting help

- Don't expect miracles. Miracles do happen but by their nature they tend to be very rare.
- Nature takes its time. If you are used to conventional medicine you may expect instant results. It may take time for any side-effects to be felt. With natural medicine the healing may be slower. Some therapists say it takes a month or two for every year that you've been ill.
- You will know the therapy is working if you feel more optimistic, more able to cope and have more energy – even if you are still getting migraine.
- Your migraines may get less serious and less frequent before they disappear altogether.
- Your migraines may come back if the cause of the underlying stress is unresolved.
- There may be long term side-effects of increased energy and creativity.

In the following chapters we'll look in turn at the natural therapies which can be helpful if you have migraine.

For how to find and choose a natural therapist see chapter 10.

CHAPTER 7

Treating your 'subtle body'

'Energy' therapies for migraine

Energy therapies treat migraine by using energy, an invisible or 'subtle' healing force (the Chinese *chi*) for its effect. In acupuncture this is done by inserting very fine needles in the body, in homoeopathy this is done through tablets or powder and in healing it is done by touch and thought.

ACUPUNCTURE

'I went on HRT and beta-blockers about four years ago to get rid of my migraine, but I was still having them about once a week and I was losing a tremendous amount of time off work. My boss suggested acupuncture to me because his mother-in-law had three or four treatments and never had a migraine again. I was very skeptical but I must admit I have had far more relief from acupuncture than anything else.

'I started having acupuncture a year ago and my migraines went from every week to ten days, then every fortnight to every three weeks. Now I have the odd headache, but there's the biggest difference in the world between ordinary headache and migraine.

'The needles don't hurt, although I felt it a couple of times when he's put one in my shoulders. It's completely relaxing. It's the only time when I'm relaxed. Normally I feel there's so many things I have to do. I used to have a cleaning lady, but she didn't do it like I do. I'm like that at the office too. I'd rather do it myself, because no-one else would do it the way I want it done. After an evening or late afternoon treatment all I want to do is go home and lie down. It's a wonderful feeling – and I usually sleep like a top. The next morning I feel great.

'At first I had acupuncture once a week, then fortnightly, and gradually built up to once every six weeks. Then I missed a couple of months in the summer because of pressure of work, but I ended up having migraines instead.

'Before I had acupuncture I was also getting a great deal of discomfort in my stomach and people said it sounded as if I had an ulcer coming. I'd also been feeling very lethargic. Now I don't have any stomach problems, I'm sleeping really well and have more energy.

'I've been putting on weight and would like to get off the beta-blockers but I tried cutting down and had a real humdinger of a migraine. I'd rather put on a bit of weight than have migraine'
– BARBARA GREEN, 50, LEGAL EXECUTIVE.

Like so many other people, Barbara Green only turned to natural medicine as a last resort. Barbara's experience is also an interesting example of acupuncture being used as a complementary therapy. In her case it complement-ed the HRT and the beta-blockers. The lethargy she com-plained of may have been one of the side-effects of the beta-blockers that the acupuncture was able to alleviate.

It's interesting that her stomach problems also cleared up – an example of the body healing itself as it gets into balance. But why was it that her boss's mother-in-law had a few treatments and never had another migraine whereas Barbara has to keep going for 'top ups'? This may be because the inner and outer stresses in her life make it difficult or impossible to *stay* in balance. The beta-blockers and HRT are still affecting her and she still expects a lot of herself.

Prescription: She should visit her doctor and discuss weaning herself off the beta-blockers and HRT – possibly with more frequent visits for acupuncture to keep herself in balance during the transition. She might also find it helpful to have counselling to help her understand and change her need for perfection.

The treatment

An acupuncture treatment starts with the acupuncturist assessing the person's basic energy-pattern and diagnosing the source of the energy imbalance by looking at your tongue and your face – and even smelling you to make an accurate diagnosis.

The most obvious way in which the practitioner makes the diagnosis is through feeling the pulse on each wrist. This enables the practitioner to feel the state of each of the 12 main 'meridians' or 'pathways' which distribute a person's 'energy' throughout the body (see figure 5). When the acupuncturist has made the diagnosis he or she will stimulate one or several of the 365 acupuncture points along the various meridians to encourage 'energy balance'. Although we associate acupuncture mainly with needles, a smouldering herb or 'moxa' (usually common mugwort) is sometimes used instead. This may be heated and attached to the needle or applied separately close to the skin. The term for this method is 'moxibustion'.

In acupuncture there's no such thing as 'migraine'. It's just one of the many signs and symptoms that tells the acupuncturist that your mind, body and emotions are out of balance. 'Anything can come from anything', so for instance an acupuncturist may find that many

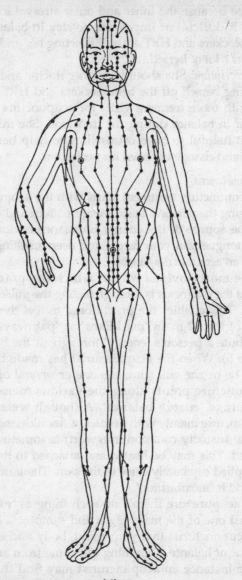

Fig. 5 The acupuncture meridians

Acupuncture points

According to the *Nan Jin*, one of the classics of Chinese medicine: 'When anger rises to the head and does not descend the liver is injured', and headaches are common in people who feel angry, or, more often, in people who don't express or resolve their anger (in other words, the anger does 'not descend'). Everyone who has migraine is different but people who have been trained in making a diagnosis in the Chinese medical system may recognize similar patterns. This is a small sample of the kind of patterns a traditional Chinese medical practitioner may notice:

- *Liver fire* is a strong pattern with a lot of angry *yang* energy in the system. The person in this pattern has very severe headaches, a red face and often feels hot. The pulse is often 'wirey' and strong, the tongue red with a coating and they would be really quite irritable with a big temper, and possibly a big appetite. Anything hot will tend to trigger a migraine: hot temper, bright sunshine, alcohol and foods with a 'heating' – *yang* – effect on the body (such as coffee, chocolate, oranges and spicy foods).

- *Liver yang* rising is a similar pattern but not as extreme or full-blown. The headaches tend to be quite bad, often on the side of the head or temple area and the cheeks may be red, or they may be quite pale. The pulse is also wirey but thin, not as strong as liver fire, and although the tongue will be red, it might only be red round the edges, with not so much coating. People in this pattern tend to be grumpy rather than angry. This pattern is also associated with such symptoms as back pain, scanty periods or dry skins. People in this pattern will tend to get migraines when they are under stress, particularly if they bottle up their anger, frustration or other emotions.

- *Phlegm picture* concerns people who tend to have more muzzy headaches, find it hard to concentrate, complain of a thick head, which is mainly in the forehead, and may have nausea. This pattern is particularly common in people who tend to be a bit overweight or have problems with their weight generally. They tend to be sluggish. This pattern is associated with the spleen and the digestive system, and is particularly associated with people who tend to get migraine when they eat the wrong things – particularly dairy foods, and cooling citrus fruits. People who are in this pattern often wake up with a bad headache (because the phlegm accumulates at night) and they tend to be pale.

people who suffer from migraine need treatment on the gall-bladder and liver meridians (see box).

Consultations

You may need to see the practitioner every two weeks for the first couple of visits, then every three or four weeks. You may find your practitioner uses both herbs and acupuncture. The first consultation lasts about one hour, follow-ups half an hour.

Research

'The sheer weight of evidence demands that acupuncture must be taken seriously as a clinical procedure of considerable value' – *The World Health Organization, 1979.*

Research in 1984 at the National Hospital for Nervous Diseases in London showed that acupuncture was more effective than conventional medicine in treating migraine and muscle-tension headaches. One patient was helped by acupuncture even though he had had depression and migraine for 50 years. In this study 59 per cent of patients benefited from acupuncture compared to only 25 per cent who had drug therapy.

But acupuncture doesn't help everyone and the fact that more than half of those in the study benefited from acupuncture is little consolation for the 41 per cent who didn't get relief.

Chinese herbs

It's only been in the past decade or so that people in the west have been trained to use Chinese herbs and the herbs themselves used to be quite difficult to find. The herbs come in different forms and practitioners vary in what they like to prescribe. The choice is usually between:

● bits of bark and root to boil at home
● concentrated powder, stirred into boiling water
● standard pills (often not powerful enough for migraines).

The skill of the practitioner is to adjust the herbs to suit the individual. People in a liver fire pattern, for example, may be given a blend containing gentian, gardenia seeds, and skull-cap root. It is a mixture that tastes very bitter and, to some, 'utterly disgusting'.

Herbs need to be taken twice a day, often for several months. The aim is to take the herbs for as long as it needs to produce an underlying change in your system. With migraine, a Chinese herbalist would expect your migraines to become milder and less frequent even though the tendency to migraine may still be there. You might tend to get a migraine after a whole day of shopping rather than just an hour. After treatment you should also feel a sense of well-being and ease.

Beware – not all the herbs are harmless It's important to go to a properly-qualified practitioner. Chinese herbal medicine is usually practised by acupuncturists who have undergone a further two year post-graduate course. In the UK contact the Register of Chinese Herbal Medicine, 9 Lawns Court, The Avenue, Wembley, Middlesex HA9 9PN.

Availability/Respectability rating
Good – not one of those therapies that's here today and gone tomorrow: the earliest acupuncture books were written in China 4,500 years ago. Worldwide there are estimated to be over three million practitioners and some pain clinics have started to use acupuncturists.

Check whether the acupuncturist is trained in Traditional Chinese Medicine (TCM), which includes Chinese diagnostic methods such as tongue and face diagnosis.

HOMOEOPATHY

'Six years ago I went to university to do a degree in English literature and my migraines got worse and worse. My hormones were dying down and I got severe flushes. I was getting left-sided headaches with nausea about three times a month and went on HRT. I was amazed by how much it helped the headaches, it was miraculous, they disappeared almost entirely. I had more energy, I could study, my hot flushes disappeared and I felt stable on a mental and emotional level.

'With the help of HRT I pushed myself to study so hard that I had a complete breakdown. I was given *amyltriptilyne* which gave me a dry mouth and seemed to put up a barrier between myself and the world. It got me functioning but I took too many tablets and ended up in hospital. My mind was so clouded, I don't even know whether it was a deliberate overdose or not. Homoeopathy had helped me in the past so I had homoeopathic treatment again and took a year off before I went back to finish my degree.

'That was a couple of years ago and I have been feeling much better. I decided to stop HRT after reading Germaine Greer and various articles. I'd been off HRT for six months when I got my first migraine in years. (For a description of this migraine, see box opposite.)

'That migraine was a turning point. It resolved several issues that needed to be looked at, I needed to decide what my priorities were. This happened

DIARY OF A MIGRAINE: Catherine Williams

Monday Emotional stress, background private worries.

Monday night/Tuesday morning Images on the TV seem unusually acute and real to my perception. Awake until about 4 am. Terrific feeling of tension and generalized pressure in my head, but no pain. Colour pictures behind my eyes of dramatic, rolling cloudscapes, like speeded up film, etc. Worries tumbling endlessly.

Tuesday No headache or pain, but feeling tired, drained and emotionally fragile. Busy day at work.

Wednesday Woke with left-sided head pain. It is always behind and above the left eye. Feeling of nausea, could easily vomit. Feel that I am falling to the left when I walk. Dropped the kettle, fortunately full of cold water. Gaps in concentration, emotionally numb. Took a pain-killer in the knowledge that it would be totally useless. *4 pm* can't write more now, the pain, sickness and dizziness getting worse. Need to be quiet. By tomorrow morning it will have gone. The pain was at its worst for about 4 hours. I lay on the settee by the fire and just allowed the pain to be. After that it began to lessen, slowly sliding away and I knew that in a few more hours it would be gone. The sensation of the pain fading made it almost enjoyable.

Thursday am As predicted, pain and nausea gone, leaving a faint shadow and a feeling of tiredness, and slowness. But I'm well and preparing to gently take up the business/busyness of life again. I feel that migraine often provides creative insights and resolutions – as though when one part of the brain is immobilised other synapses can open.

It was after this particular episode that Catherine decided to resign from her part-time job and concentrate on her degree. She also had her first experience of giving someone spiritual healing.

over a period of four days. It started the day before the pain started, then there was the day of intense pain and a couple of days recovering when I made decisions and had insights about what I was doing with my life.

'My homoeopath has just given me the homoeopathic remedy *natrum muriaticum* for my shoulder and neck. I get all stiff and knotted up, it's difficult to get comfortable at night. I also take vitamin E for hot flushes and I find that two a day keeps them at bay' – CATHERINE WILLIAMS, 54, RETIRED MEDICAL SECRETARY DOING A DEGREE IN ENGLISH LITERATURE.

Migraine may be viewed as the body's best way of balancing itself – it's 'time off' from external stimulation. It's not our *symptoms* that cause dis-ease, its our *dis-ease* that creates the symptoms. In Catherine's case, a homoeopath might say she needed to take time off, to take her degree more slowly. This was an unconscious feeling her body tried to communicate through her migraines. She overrode the safety signal of the migraine so her 'vital force' had to find another way of sending her the same message – hence her breakdown.

As she got better and recovered from her mental collapse she could think more clearly and decided to come off HRT which may have been suppressing her migraines. Interestingly enough, six months after stopping HRT she experienced her first migraine in years. She also experienced the healing effect the migraine itself can have. The migraine helped her to re-examine her life: she resigned her job and after years of denying her potential as a healer she allowed herself to give someone healing and discovered her innate ability to channel and see healing energy.

Having recovered from her migraine, Catherine's 'vital force' is giving her stiff neck and shoulders, signals that she is still stressed (but not at such a deep level as in the middle of a migraine). Her body is saying that it needs a new homoeopathic remedy, and the remedy that was prescribed for her is a common remedy for people with a tendency to get migraine (see p. 84).

Many homoeopaths believe there's a certain logic in the way people get ill, and the way we get well. When Catherine's migraines were suppressed she became more ill and had a breakdown. When she stopped suppressing her migraine with HRT she had another migraine – and now she is experiencing shoulder and neck tension which is a milder physical expression of the tension in her life (see box 'Law of Cure' below).

The homoeopathic 'Law of Cure'

We tend to get ill – and get well – in a logical order. Minor health problems tend to be only skin deep, major ones can be life-threatening. If your migraine disappears but you get high blood pressure, this is a sign that your general state of health is deteriorating. Migraine isn't life-threatening, high blood pressure can be. Perhaps the best known example of this healing logic is *eczema*, which can be a very distressing skin complaint. But it's only on the surface of your body. If this is suppressed it can result in *asthma*, which can be life-threatening. If asthma is cured it can result in a return of the original eczema.

When we get into balance the worst problems get better first. Homoeopaths and other natural therapists expect you to feel better mentally and emotionally before you feel physically better. After all, there's no point in having a healthy body if you feel so miserable you commit suicide. As your health improves your illnesses should become more and more minor.

The homoeopathic interview

The first consultation usually lasts between one and two hours. The homoeopath may need this long to get enough information to understand you well enough so that he or she can decide on the most appropriate remedy for you. You may be asked about:

- past medical history
- foods you like/dislike
- weather and temperature you like/dislike
- specific fears
- emotional and mental state
- things that make you feel better/worse.

Once you've been given the remedy the homoeopath will probably want to see you again in four to six weeks to see how you are responding. Follow-up appointments tend to be briefer, lasting about half an hour.

Homoeopathic remedy patterns

Everyone who suffers from migraine experiences it in their own unique way, so a homoeopathic remedy that helps one person might not help someone else. There are over 2,000 homoeopathic remedies to choose from (involving a variety of plants, minerals and other substances) so selecting the right one to suit the individual is both an art and a science. The art is to discover which particular homoeopathic pattern fits each individual person most precisely, and the science is the experience and knowledge that homoeopaths have built up over the 200 years since the therapy was first developed.

For example, there are over 50 'common' headache remedies to choose from, and it's obviously not possible to describe each one in this particular book. A look at the following two remedy patterns illustrates that it can be quite difficult to differentiate between them – and this task is best left to experts:

Case 1: Jean's story (the calcarea carbonicum pattern)
'After my first migraine when I was 23 I had them about once or twice a year until my menopause when I started to get them every six to eight weeks. The headache is

always left-sided and it's a dull throbbing pain. There's a tremendous pressure and I used to bang my head on the bedhead just to experience another kind of pain. I was also violently sick. But when it was all over I felt absolutely marvellous, as if I could skip over mountains.

'Right from the beginning the homoeopathic remedy stopped me being physically sick. The migraines were also less frequent and went from every six weeks to two months to every three to four months, then every four to five months and the last one was nine months ago. But it doesn't knock me out, I'm not prostrate. It's like a shadow. I don't feel like breakfast, I don't feel right. It's a niggle. I'm not suffering but if I try to do mental work I know I would be very slow or make mistakes. When I had full migraine I couldn't use my mind at all, I couldn't think.

'It's such a relief to have conquered migraine. I feel so much better. I have wonderful peak days when I feel so well I feel marvellous. I read about my homoeopathic type, *calcarea carbonica*, which has been described as 'Scrooge-cold, as closed, secretive and self-contained as an oyster'. I identify with a lot of that description and especially love the idea of me being a pearl inside an oyster' – JEAN STUBBS, 67, NOVELIST.

Homoeopaths view symptoms as the body's efforts to remain in balance with the stress of living. These stresses can be internal, or external, and often both. Jean's migraines got more frequent when she was approaching menopause. She had also experienced 'the worst year of her life' in the long hot summer of 1976 when she had a huge tax bill and couldn't get her books published. She was battling against trying to be 'too good' and found it difficult to put herself first.

After three years of homoeopathic treatment she now has no migraines at all and has not needed to take a rem-

edy for over a year. Occasionally she gets a feeling of a
slight headache or queasiness which she can ignore. She
feels well and says she has more energy now than for the
past 20 years.

The homoeopathic remedy *calcarea carbonica* is taken
from the middle layer of the oyster shell. The main
theme which is common to people who need this remedy is that they can't cope with stress and feel out of control. Like the oyster, they need a shell to act as a buffer
between their inner life and their environment. They
tend to be reserved, withdrawn and self-reliant and will
often become ill after prolonged effort to overcome
stress.

Other reasons for choosing *calcarea carbonica* for Jean
are:

- *Her personality* she is self-contained and independent.
- *Her emotions* she cries easily and openly in sympathy
  with other people, but she is not open about her own
  emotions. She has to fight against bottling everything
  up.
- *Her fears* as a child she was 'extraordinarily full of
  fear' and was frightened of thunder and lightning,
  ghosts, cows, and spiders. She was terrified of things
  that happened suddenly. For example, she would
  jump if a door slammed. These fears are typical of
  someone who is in 'a *calcarea* remedy pattern'.
- *The migraines themselves* her migraines were better
  once she could vomit. She could go to sleep within two
  minutes of vomiting because the pain was so much
  less and when she woke up the pain was usually gone
  altogether.
- *Other physical symptoms* Jean had flaking nails where
  the end of the nail separates in layers and also had
  breast cysts. Both the breast cysts and the flaky nails
  are typical calcarea symptoms.

• *Other factors* Jean is a very chilly person, has to wear bedsocks at night and extreme cold makes her face hurt, especially her forehead and nose. She also puts on weight very easily and likes soft-boiled eggs.

Jean was given *calcarea* to bring her whole energy system into balance. It would not have helped her when she was in the middle of an acute attack. *Belladonna* might have helped her in an acute attack because she couldn't bear light or company, but it wouldn't have prevented her from suffering any more attacks.

Case 2 Susan's story (the natrum muriaticum *pattern)*
'I went to see the homoeopath about my vaginal thrush. I didn't expect he could do anything about my migraine because I knew it was stress-related. My migraines started after my separation which ended in divorce. Sometimes I could bash my head against the wall with the pain. The slightest noise was deafening, like a thundering and hammering in my head. I don't know how I coped with them.

'The first homoeopathic remedy back-fired, my thrush was even worse and it appeared in my mouth. My homoeopath changed the prescription and the thrush got better and so did my headaches. As an added bonus I now have more confidence. Before I would worry about the slightest remark, now I might worry but only for an hour, not for a whole day like I used to. Now I only get a migraine for a very good reason.

'A few months ago I had a bad one and I knew it was emotional. I was holding back from saying what I needed to say. When I realized what was happening I dealt with the problem. I deal with problems a lot better now. I knew the migraines were stress-related and I still get them, but they are not nearly as bad as they used to be and they don't last very long. I don't have thrush any more either.' – SUSAN JONES, 55, MANAGING DIRECTOR OF INDUSTRIAL COMPLEX.

One of the interesting things about Susan's experience is that for ten years before she got migraine she suffered from severe indigestion with wind and belching and a dull pain in the pit of her stomach. These disappeared when her migraine started and came back when her migraines got better. At one time she would have a bout of indigestion for three or four weeks and be clear for six weeks and then it would come back again (see box 'Law of Cure', page 79).

After three years of homoeopathy even the indigestion has gradually subsided. She only gets the occasional headache and says she's able to talk about her problems more now. She also has more energy. It has been two years since she last needed a remedy.

The 'English remedy'

Some homoeopaths think that *natrum muriaticum* is the commonest migraine remedy in Britain today. This is because the remedy works best on those with the typical 'English' personality. That is, on those people who are rather sensitive and reserved. They tend to be hardworking perfectionists and are easily hurt, with a fear of being rejected.

Someone who is in a *natrum muriaticum* pattern can have any kind of headache, but will often get some form of visual aura such as zig-zag lines before the headache starts and nausea, maybe with vomiting, when the headache is severe. People in a *natrum muriaticum* pattern find it very difficult to put on weight and if they are ill they lose weight very quickly. This is the opposite of people like Jean Stubbs who are in a *calcarea carbonicum* pattern who put on weight very easily.

Most people are irritable and want to be alone during a migraine but in the person who is in a long-term *natrum muriaticum* pattern, the desire for solitude will be more pronounced than the irritability of someone in a *calcarea carbonicum* pattern.

Getting worse before you get better

Like Susan Jones, you might find that you get worse if you are given the wrong homoeopathic remedy. However even if it's the right remedy you may still feel worse before you get better. Some people experience an 'aggravation', some people don't. You may experience a particularly severe migraine and never have one again. Or, more likely, the migraines may become milder and increasingly less frequent.

How quickly will you get better?

If it's the right homoeopathic remedy acute illnesses can respond very quickly – but the longer you've had it the longer it may take to cure it.

Homoeopaths estimate that it takes about a month for every year you've had the problem – so, for example, it could take some 20 months before you are migraine-free if you've had migraines for 20 years. On the other hand, your body may respond to the remedy more quickly, or more slowly. Also some remedies are faster-acting than others.

If the homoeopath has found the right remedy for you, you may start to feel better quite quickly in the beginning. Even though your physical symptoms are unchanged you may feel that you can cope better with your illness and have more energy.

Why isn't homoeopathy used more?

If it is so successful it is reasonable to ask why it isn't used more. The answer is it takes a great deal of time, study and practice to become a good homoeopath. It is difficult and time-consuming to learn how to recognize the subtle differences between all the different remedy patterns. When homoeopaths first qualify they may be able to help only some 10-20 per cent of patients. After ten years they might have enough experience to be able to find the right remedy for maybe 70-80 per cent of them. Some people claim it takes over 20 years to become a homoeopathic 'master' – but even after a life-time's experience the best practitioner is unlikely to be able to find the right remedy for everybody.

Will homoeopathy be able to help you?

Yes – but only if the homoeopath finds the right remedy, and depending also on how you manage to change and what new insights you bring to your condition. Good homoeopathic treatment helps you understand both yourself and your migraine.

Research

By definition the right homoeopathic remedy will cure migraine, the wrong one won't. This means it's not homoeopathy itself on trial but the skill of the practition-er. A particular homoeopathic remedy will work well only if it's the correct remedy for *that particular individ-ual*. (If the wrong remedy is taken repeatedly it may make the condition worse.)

Nevertheless several studies have shown that homoeopathy is effective in treating migraine. For exam-ple, in one study in Italy involving 60 patients there was a significant reduction in intensity, frequency and dura-tion of the migraines in the homoeopathically treated group compared with a group that was only given a placebo.

In another study in Britain treatments by a homoeo-pathic doctor who used homoeopathic remedies, exclu-sion diets and homoeopathic neutralizers for food and house dust mite allergies were analyzed. This showed that out of 54 patients treated for migraine over a period of 18 months 43 did well and found improvement in their symptoms in the four weeks after the first consulta-tion.

Availability/respectability rating

Variable. In Britain it's respectable enough for the National Health Service and for the Royal Family and there are a respectable enough number of qualified practitioners – both medical and non-medical – practising it. Doctors in Glasgow are learning about it and the John Moore University in Liverpool starts teaching it to doctors in 1994. In the UK most practising homoeopaths are not doctors. Some are, but the majority who aren't call themselves 'professional homoeopaths'. In Europe as a whole, though, homoeopathy is most widely practised by doctors, particularly in France and Germany, with growing numbers in eastern Europe (because it's cheap and it works). Outside Europe homoeopathy is practised, and accepted, increasingly in countries like Australia, New Zealand, South Africa and the USA. It has been banned in the US state of South Carolina but is available in other states.

HEALING

'I had my first migraine when I was 19 and left home to live in London. I had Mondays off, and used to wander around Hyde Park Corner and several times I was suddenly struck by violent migraine. I can put them to one side if there's a crisis, but when I relax afterwards I get a blinding headache and I'm violently sick. At one stage I was getting them almost every week. It was awful.

'When I was violently sick it gave me some relief but it was only temporary. When my stomach is totally empty and the migraine has finally subsided I feel uplifted. I feel like a weight has lifted from my shoulders and I'm more able to cope.

I tried homoeopathy but it didn't do anything.

Then an exclusion diet but couldn't find anything that brought on the migraine. Chiropractic seemed to help but the migraines came back after a few months. An osteopath said he couldn't help. Wearing glasses to correct a slight stigmatism didn't have any effect either.

'Daily beta-blockers helped for a while, but then the effect seemed to wear off and my migraines came back. My most recent discovery is that if I can take an aspirin and sit quietly at the first warning sign I can avoid a full-blown migraine. But once the migraine is under way and I have been sick nothing can stop it.

'Since September I've seen several spiritual healers and received very good help. I'm usually aware of warmth and a deep feeling of inner calm. Sometimes if I have a deep inner conflict the healing will bring them to the surface and I may get an insight about what to do. I feel that in the past I've been controlled by "shoulds" and "oughts" and carry on until I drop. I'm trying to be more sensible.

'Healing really made a difference. In the four months since I've been having spiritual healing I've only had one migraine, but it was only mild, not devastating like it usually is. I feel much more responsible for my own health now. My depression has lifted and I've stopped taking my anti-depressants' – MICHAEL SLAUGHTER, 48.

Michael tried practically every treatment going before he turned to spiritual healing. So far he has had good results, but the interesting thing is that he now takes more responsibility for his own health. He is starting to recognize that he generates some of his own stress, and healing has given him the energy and optimism to tackle his inner conflicts. He has also started meditating.

The treatment

What happens when you go for healing very much depends on the personal style of the healer and the particular form of healing they practise. For example, a nurse practising 'Therapeutic Touch' may have a different approach than someone who practises 'spiritual healing'. However, the treatment often follows a fairly consistent pattern:

● Healers start by preparing themselves through thought, meditation or prayer. This doesn't usually take very long.

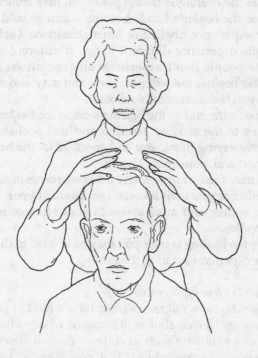

Fig. 6 A healer at work

- Healers may then put their hands on your shoulders or head (or they may put their hands a few inches away from your body: *see figure 6*. At this point the healer is making contact with your 'energy', and may be 'asking permission' or praying for the healing to take place.

- Healers may then pass their hands down your spine and/or touch different parts of your body. Again, this may be a physical 'laying-on-of-hands' or they may keep their hands a few inches away from your body and work on your energy body (also known as the 'aura').

- While the healing is taking place you may sometimes notice the healer's hands become warm or cold, you may experience tingling or other sensations. Different people experience different things at different times. Some people don't experience any sensations at all during healing but still get relief. You may also notice that you feel increasingly relaxed.

- Towards the end of the healing session the healer may return to the starting position and will probably be silently saying thank you and goodbye to 'the healing energy' and your energy body.

- You may then want to spend a few moments in silence together as you both become less aware of your 'energetic bodies' and more aware of your separate physical bodies.

- After the healing is over you may be invited to discuss your experiences during the healing.

A healer's view of migraine

'People who have migraines often have a kind of jangly, tense energy. It feels similar to someone who has had too much of a stimulant such as coffee. I think it affects the whole energy system but if it is concentrated on any single energy centre it would be the brow and/or the solar plexus.

'People who suffer from epilepsy also have very tense energy like people with migraine, but their nervous system gets even more overloaded before the seizure. Migraine seems to act as a safety cut-out on an overloaded system. Healing helps to relieve excessive stress in the nervous system and also it often helps us to relax and process information better. It helps you to do whatever you need to do to heal yourself. Healing works on many levels simultaneously. It can help you spontaneously to gain insight into what's happening and what you need to do about it' – Jessica Macbeth, healer, founder of the Order of the Ascending Spirit in the USA and head of its UK branch.

Research

Perhaps surprisingly there is more research evidence to support the efficacy of healing than there is for all the other complementary therapies combined, with the exception of hypnosis.

For example, in one trial on people suffering from tension headaches randomly allocated to 'placebo touch' or Therapeutic Touch. The people who had Therapeutic Touch noticed sensations of tingling, warmth and relaxation during the healing – even though they were not told what to expect. The placebo intervention did reduce headache pain but wasn't as effective and didn't last as long as the Therapeutic Touch. It has also been shown that more experienced healers have produced significantly greater reductions in anxiety than inexperienced healers.

Availability/Respectability rating

Good. In the US there are tens of thousands of nurses who have been trained in 'Therapeutic Touch' as well as thousands of lay-people who have been trained as healers. In some states, and in many other countries such as Germany, it is illegal to practise spiritual healing as a profession: you must be licensed in another therapy or be authorized by a church.

In the UK there are no restrictions on the right to practise. Over 8,000 healers are members of organizations that belong to the Confederation of Healing Organizations and some estimates put the number of practising healers in Britain at more than 30,000 and this number is rising. Healers are increasingly being used in doctors' surgeries and in pain clinics attached to hospitals.

CHAPTER 8

Treating your body

Physical therapies for migraine

'One day, when about ten years old, I suffered from a headache. I made a swing of my father's plow-line between two trees – but my head hurt too much to make swinging comfortable so I let the rope down to about eight or ten inches off the ground, threw the end of a blanket on it, and I lay down on the ground and used the rope for a swinging pillow. Thus I lay stretched on my back, with my neck across the rope. Soon I became easy and went to sleep, got up in a little while with my headache gone. As I knew nothing of anatomy at this time I took no thought of how a rope could stop headache and the sick stomach which accompanied it. After that discovery I roped my neck whenever I felt one of those spells coming on. I followed that treatment for twenty years before the wedge of reason reached my brain, and I could see that I had suspended the action of the great occipital nerves, and given harmony to the flow of the arterial blood to and through the veins, and ease was the effect, as the reader can see' – ANDREW TAYLOR STILL, FOUNDER OF OSTEOPATHY, FROM HIS AUTOBIOGRAPHY.

Migraine is sometimes the result of a mechanical problem – and it is worth checking this out with one of the physical therapists such as an osteopath, chiropractor, physiotherapist, massage therapist – or even your dentist.

DENTISTRY

Your dentist may be able to help you if you suffer from migraine because you clench your jaw. The medical name for this phenomena is *temporomandibular joint dysfunction*, or TMJ pain. The TMJ is the joint located in front of the ear connecting the upper and lower jaws. Pain from the nerves supplying this area can radiate to include the side of the face, head and neck. Dentists have had considerable success in helping people with migraine by correcting their 'bite', the way in which the two jaws meet when you bite. Your dentist may also recommend that you see an osteopath or chiropractor as well as use some form of relaxation and stress management technique.

If there's nothing wrong with your bite you may still be clenching your jaw in your sleep. Wearing a 2mm-thick splint over the back teeth at night may help according to recent research. It found that 40 per cent of sufferers reduced the incidence of migraine by two-thirds when they wore the splint.

Café-owner Jenny Gale accidentally discovered the connection between jaws and migraine when she had her wisdom teeth out:

> 'About eighteen months ago I was having terrible migraines about twice a fortnight. I had all my wisdom teeth out and my migraines stopped instantly. I've had a lot of repressed anger, I was clenching my jaw a lot and after I had my wisdom teeth out, I made a conscious effort not to. After I had my wisdom teeth out, my relationship improved and I was able to express myself a lot better. I think it was all connected to my jaw.'

Dental work can cause migraine as well as cure it, and some osteopaths feel that the trauma of dentistry can

affect the positioning of the bones in the head and neck
and this can lead to migraine. Therapists who specialize
in manipulation to correct such 'imbalances' are mainly
chiropractors, osteopaths and physiotherapists.

MANIPULATION

Migraine can often be traced back to 'mechanical insults'
such as a whiplash injury in a car, a rugby injury, a fall
on the head, or simply knocking your head on a cup-
board door. In Elizabeth's case her migraine started
when she had children:

> 'I'm 32 years old, happily married with two boys
> aged 9 and 4 and my migraines started after I had
> my first child. At first I got left-sided headaches
> every two or three months, which lasted a day or
> two just before my periods. After I had my second
> son they got much worse and more frequent. I got
> them every month, just before my period, lasting
> two or three days, when I had to stay in bed because
> the nausea and vomiting was so bad. I had a lot of
> lower back pain during both my pregnancies, but
> I'm generally quite healthy, if a little bit overweight.
> I try not to eat fatty foods or junk food, I don't
> smoke or drink and go to keep-fit class every week.
> I find that looking after the two boys is quite stress-
> ful. I had some osteopathic treatment once a week
> for a few weeks and my migraines have stopped,
> and I seem to be coping better with the boys now.'

Like Elizabeth, many women realize that their migraines
started – or got worse – when they had children. Perhaps
this isn't surprising because pregnancy makes the pelvis
tilt to cope with the extra weight and this can put your
whole spine out of balance. In Elizabeth's case an

osteopath was able to help her spine to return to its pre-pregnancy balance, but the effective therapy could as easily have been chiropractic or physiotherapy.

CHIROPRACTIC

Availability/respectability rating
High, in most countries. Chiropractic is the largest primary healthcare profession in the Western world after medicine and dentistry and its practitioners are highly trained and tightly controlled. In most countries, especially North America, it is easily the single largest 'natural therapy' practised. In the US there is one chiropractor for every two physical therapists (known as physiotherapists in the UK). In the UK, by contrast, physiotherapists outnumber chiropractors by 20 to one.

Research
In 1990 the *British Medical Journal* reported the results of the UK Medical Research Council's eight year multi-centre trial comparing chiropractic treatment to outpatient management of patients with acute and chronic mechanical low back pain. Chiropractic treatment was found to be more effective in clinical and economic terms both in the short and long term. The journal, one of the world's most prestigious medical journals, recommended that chiropractic be introduced into British hospitals for treating low back pain.

OSTEOPATHY

Availability/respectability rating
Good. In July 1993 an Act of Parliament established osteopathy as the first 'natural therapy' to be recognized

by law in Britain and the General Osteopathic Council, to regulate the practice of all osteopaths, is expected to start work in 1995. In the USA osteopaths are already recognized by being all medical doctors (it is a post-graduate training). In Britain there are about 3000 osteopaths in practice as opposed to only about 500 chiropractors. In other countries there are fewer osteopaths than chiropractors.

Research

Osteopaths have carried out surprisingly little research but in Britain there have been a couple of recent studies which showed it can help migraine.

What's the difference between osteopaths and chiropractors?

Not a lot, except in America where osteopaths are medical doctors and chiropractors are not. Elsewhere they both tend to be 'non-medical' practitioners in the sense they operate outside the medical profession. In practice, osteopaths and chiropractors both use manipulation to correct 'imbalances' to the joints and muscles of the body (the musculo-skeletal system), particularly the spine. But with chiropractors the 'adjustments' tend to be more vigorous. Chiropractors are also more likely to use x-ray in their initial diagnosis whereas osteopaths rely more on what they see, hear and feel when they make their diagnosis.

Some osteopaths practise cranial osteopathy, or cranio-sacral therapy, which deals with the bones of the head. This specialist form of osteopathy is particularly suitable for treating migraine if it has developed as a result of a fall, accident or where major dental work has changed the alignment of the 'bite'.

PHYSIOTHERAPY/PHYSICAL THERAPY

Availability/respectability rating

Good. In most Western countries it is a state-recognized and regulated profession allied to conventional medicine, with strict standards and controls. In the US there are twice as many physical therapists as chiropractors. In Britain physical therapists are known as physiotherapists and there are 25,000 registered, practising both privately and in the public health sector.

Research

There is about as much research as in osteopathy to show its benefit in migraine.

OTHER PHYSICAL THERAPIES

'I had my first migraine in September 1988 at the Glasgow Garden Festival, but I've only had three since then. I wouldn't want any more. I use a mixture my aromatherapy massage therapist made up for me. I also have massage about once a month. I wish I could afford to have it more often, it's wonderful. Migraine is different from an ordinary headache: I see coloured lines and I can't see out of the bottom half of my eyes. It's awful. If I can massage myself then it's alright, it will go away. If it develops I can't bear anyone to touch me. I have to be alone. I get pain in the back of my neck and I feel like I want to be sick and I have to lie down'
– WILMA.

The fact that Wilma has only had three migraines since 1988 may be luck. But it may also be due to the fact that she has regular massage for her tense muscles, and uses aromatherapy when a migraine threatens.

Much of the pain of migraine comes from chronically

tight muscles. These may be the muscles in the neck, the upper back, the skull or the muscles which control the jaw. Some people find that it helps to have regular massage to relieve the tension in the muscles, but the benefits of massage will be short-lived if the underlying problems are not dealt with.

Tense muscles may be the result of emotional stress or trauma and may be helped by less well-known therapies such as 'Rolfing', bioenergetics, dance therapy, reflexology (including its latest hi-tech version 'Vacuflex therapy') and other 'bodywork' specialities that can help you to release the emotions that may be locked into your tight muscles.

Tense muscles can also be the result of bad posture. An occupational therapist can tell you whether you need to change the way you sit at your desk (perhaps you need a different chair) and how you sit when you drive. You can also improve your posture with lessons from a teacher of the 'Alexander Technique', a way of helping you sit, stand, lie (see figure 7) and move in an easy and stress-free way .

Exercise can also loosen muscle-tension and some people find yoga particularly helpful. A survey of students and teachers who suffered from migraine found

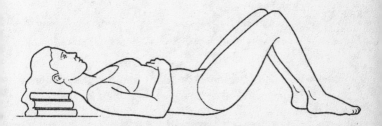

Fig. 7 An Alexander Technique relaxation exercise

shown improvements and after a year three-quarters had. However some people find that they actually feel worse after yoga. If that happens to you, tell your instructor who may be able to advise you. Your instructor may suggest that you need to change your practice (or perhaps change the way you position your head).

Summary

The physical therapies work if the root of the migraine has a mechanical cause. But good results may not last, particularly if there are more severe underlying problems that the physical therapy doesn't address. For example, an osteopath, chiropractor or massage therapist can free your neck and shoulders – but if your body wants to duck away and hide every time your boss comes in your neck and shoulders will quickly become tense and tight again.

At some point in the process of dealing with your migraines you may reach the conclusion that no matter what you do nothing works – and even if it does work it doesn't seem to work for very long. Why should this happen, and what can you do about it? Read the next chapter.

CHAPTER 9

Treating your mind and emotions

Therapies for how you think and feel

If you have:

- Tried lots of different therapies and are getting nowhere;
- Know you should quit smoking, drinking, drugs, coffee - but can't;
- Know you should avoid chocolate, cheese or some other food, but you eat it before you remember your migraine;
- Know you shouldn't work hard - but do anyway;
- Tried lots of therapies that don't work - or if they do work, they don't work for long;

don't panic. It's time you got help from a good counsellor, hypnotherapist or psychotherapist, the kind of help that will help you understand what your body is trying to tell your mind and emotions. Your unconscious mind may need something that only migraine can provide.

Is your migraine helping you avoid life?

When you have a migraine you're often forced to say 'no': no, I can't do this perfectly, no I can't go to this meeting, no I can't talk to my husband/wife/boss, take an exam, finish a project, have fun. Whatever it is, it's your body saying 'no'. Even if you manage to force yourself and 'soldier on' you're not really all there. Part of you is dealing with the migraine.

You probably think that none of this applies to you. You're right. Your conscious mind is perfectly happy with the way things are. It's your unconscious that is having so much difficulty trying to make itself heard through your body. Most of us have problems deciphering what our unconscious is trying to tell us – which is where counselling, hypnotherapy or psychotherapy can be helpful.

Cognitive therapy

The way we feel affects the way we think, and the way we think affects the way we feel. So what happens to migraine when we talk about it in different ways? Does the language we use make migraine easier or more difficult to deal with? Does the language you use empower you – or empower your migraine? For example, how do you describe migraine? Do you talk about migraine 'attacks' and migraine 'triggers'? Do you think of yourself as a migraine 'victim'? How do you feel when you realize that migraine has the power to *trigger an attack*? Does it make you feel like a *victim*?

You may have noticed that this book tries to avoid the word 'attack' and talks about episodes and incidents caused or set off (not triggered), and there are no victims or patients – only people. This is not trivializing migraine but empowering *you* rather than your migraine. This approach is called 'cognitive restructuring'. It's been used successfully to treat depression and other psychological problems and has been found to be useful in helping people in chronic pain. The idea is to identify and then rewrite your 'internal scripts'. Thoughts such as 'I'm never going to get rid of this migraine' or 'I can't take any more' are understandable but unhelpful. Cognitive restructuring revolves around identifying negative thoughts and feelings and learning how to change them.

In one study, people with recurrent tension headaches who had been trained in cognitive restructuring had a 43-100 per cent improvement in their headaches. So far this has not been tested on migraine but the Pain Evaluation and Treatment Institute of the University of Pittsburgh School of Medicine has found cognitive therapy useful for migraine-sufferers when it is combined with relaxation training and biofeedback.

Problem-solving

I am a journalist on a monthly magazine and I usually get a migraine as soon as the deadline is over and the articles have all gone to the printers. I know I drink too much coffee but it's the only way I can cope with the mounting pressure just before deadline. My migraines were getting so bad that I realized I needed to do something about it. I went to a pain clinic who helped me realize what was happening and they encouraged me to try biofeedback, to have massage in the week before my deadline and to stop drinking coffee.

'It didn't work. Then I realized that my editor had been leaning on me. I'd been producing twice as many articles as my colleagues so no wonder I felt pressurized. I talked about the problem to my editor who actually thought I thrived on adrenalin. Now she realizes I'm not a complete superwoman she's not expecting quite so much of me, and I've started to turn down assignments when I feel overloaded' – JEAN SMITH.

It wasn't enough for Jean to identify her stress pattern and try to change her reactions to the stress. She had to find ways of solving the underlying problem – over-work. This form of therapy is known as 'problem-solving' and it is often used with cognitive restructuring. As you identify situations that seem to bring on your migraine you may need help in solving the problems that arise in those situations. In Jean's case she recognized that her migraines started after her deadlines, but she needed to solve the problem of being given (and accepting) too much work.

Just because Jean found a way of solving her problem, doesn't mean that the migraine was her 'fault'. No one wants to get migraine. You may think that your problems aren't as simple as Jean's – and you may be right.

The 'monkey' puzzle

If you're the sort of person who's always very busy you might find this story about monkeys useful and informative – or you may be so distracted by other people's monkeys that you haven't got enough time to read it. Let's see...

Imagine your problems and responsibilities are monkeys – any type, any size: big ones, little ones, some you can't get rid of. You need to look after them, clean up after them, feed them and as soon as you turn your back they're breeding like, well, monkeys. You've got monkeys on your back, your shoulders and head. They're everywhere.

Of course other people have monkeys too, and they'd like to give them to you. But stop and think. Do you really want more monkeys? The trick is to recognize what's happening, be firm and say: NO MORE MONKEYS. Keep your problems to yourself.

Lawyers are professional monkey-keepers. They specialize in other people's problems. Is your job keeping a primate house? Next time someone comes to you with a problem, think about it. Is it their monkey or your monkey? If it's their monkey, do you really want to take it from them? Haven't you got enough monkeys of your own? If so, don't be afraid to put up your hand and say 'no more.'

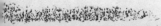

Hypnotherapy

'I look drunk and I can't think straight, the migraines themselves are agony and the rest of the time I'm irritable and get depressed. When I went to see the hypnotherapist I remembered my sister being jealous of me. When I was little she used to get me into trouble, she still does. On my third visit I remembered waiting in fear for my drunken violent stepfather to come home. After a few visits my migraine stopped, my vision improved and I wasn't so hysterical with the children. Under hypnosis I remembered what happened 30 years ago when I was 13 and my father died. I gradually realized that I got my headaches from my mother. She worries so much and treats me as if I were still a child. She didn't want me to have a white wedding and refused to speak to me. After that session I had a headache for six days, but at least it wasn't a migraine. After that last headache I have started to get slightly itchy skin. I still have trouble saying no, but what my mother says has stopped worrying me. After 20 sessions my migraine had gone, my itching had gone and I'd found out a lot about myself'
– DIANA, 43, MOTHER OF THREE.

Diana's experience with her drunken step-father shows that she may have developed an ability to be sensitive to her surroundings so that she could sense when her step-father was about to behave unpredictably. These circumstances may have unconsciously encouraged her to have a very active or 'open' reticular activating system (see 'All about the brain', chapter 1, p. 14).

As Diana resolved her unconscious irritation with her mother her migraines improved but she developed a physical irritation – her itchy skin. Her skin stopped itching when she stopped being anxious about her mother and learned how to say no. Migraine is the body's way of saying 'no'. In Diana's case, she couldn't cope with her children or her mother. Her migraine was her body's way of saying 'leave me alone'.

Before she had hypnotherapy Diana was totally unaware of what her body was trying to tell her. Consciously she wanted to be a good daughter and mother. It was her unconscious that had the problem. A good therapist will help you to identify what your unconscious is saying, to unravel what your body is trying to tell your mind.

Hypnotherapy worked for Diana because she was prepared to find out about herself and face up to her repressed feelings. Hypnotherapy uses hypnosis to help you to remember your repressed feelings and therapy helps you to deal with what you remember. But you don't necessarily need to see a hypnotherapist for this. You may find that your feelings are bubbling up close to the surface and a few simple counselling sessions may help you.

You may even become aware of the root of your difficulty (and how to resolve it) when you are relaxing or meditating (see chapter 5 'Activating your own healing system'). Self-hypnosis may be useful here.

Discovering what your unconscious feels about you and your migraines is the opposite to the kind of hypnosis where you are hypnotized and told that you will not have migraine any more. This can sometimes mask the underlying problem and create fresh symptoms. Your unconscious may agree not to have migraine, but you may develop something such as depression instead. This kind of hypnosis is sometimes used to help people stop smoking and it can work quite well. However some people find that although it helps them stop smoking they find another destructive way of dealing with their problems such as eating or drinking too much.

Self-hypnosis

Self-hypnosis is simply a combination of relaxation and imagery. It can be an effective form of pain relief, but you can also use relaxation and imagery to help you gain a better understanding about your migraine. For example, if your migraine were an animal what kind of an animal would it be? What does that animal want from you? Can you give your migraine what it wants? The first answer that comes into your head will be the right answer for you.

'I always feel that my migraine is my body being angry with me. The first animal I thought of was a tiger but I tried to ignore it. He wanted me to leave my partner but I'm frightened. Tigers are quite brave, aren't they? I never thought of myself as a tiger but I did want to break up my relationship a few months ago and was too scared. I ended up with an awful migraine and my migraines have got worse as my relationship has deteriorated' – CAROLINE S.

Your migraine may be a different animal: a cat that has been 'overwhelmed' or run over by a car, a donkey that refuses to budge. Different people have different migraines – and different animals. What's your animal? What does it tell you about your migraine? You may need help with this and many counsellors and therapists use this kind of imagery work to help people to help themselves.

Respectability rating

Varied. Hypnosis is still trying to shake off its showbiz image where people are hypnotized into doing silly things. But it is increasingly used by medical doctors. The doctor who won the 1993 'Migraine Doctor of the Year Award' in Britain teaches self-hypnosis to people with migraine. The relatively new therapy 'Neuro-Linguistic Programming' (NLP), in which your subconscious is 'reprogrammed', is based on the principles of hypnosis.

Research

Hypnosis has been subjected to more controlled trials than any other natural therapy. In one study, for example, children between six and twelve years old given drugs (*propranolol*), placebos and self-hypnosis for recurring headaches found that the number of headaches per child was roughly the same same for the placebo period and during the drug treatment period (13.3 headaches and 14.9 respectively) – but less than half (5.8) during the self-hypnosis period. Children were taught a progressive relaxation exercise followed by focusing on some pleasant image of their own choosing. The children were told to practise for ten minutes twice a day.

CHAPTER 10

How to find and choose a natural therapist

Tips and guidelines for seeking out reliable help

Natural therapy is not organized in the neat and uniform way conventional medicine is and finding and choosing a natural therapist who is right for you is therefore not as simple as contacting your local family doctor.

There is only one ideal way to find the right therapist – conventional or natural – and that is to ask, ask, and ask again. If three people have been helped by the same practitioner he or she is likely to be able to help you as well. Ask your friends, family, colleagues and acquaintances. Can they recommend a good therapist? Personal recommendation is always the best guide.

If you don't know a relative or friend who can recommend someone your local healthfood shop or alternative bookshop might be helpful. People who work there tend to be unbiased and knowledgeable about which therapists are really good because they are at the centre of a network of people who use alternatives.

Failing that ask your family doctor or migraine clinic if they can recommend a natural therapist who has had success in treating migraine. Some migraine clinics have their own natural therapists.

If you know a natural therapist socially you may not want to see him or her professionally, but you can ask them to recommend someone else. Natural therapists tend to know each other, and will hear clients singing the praises of therapists who have helped them (or moaned about therapists who didn't.).

Your local natural health centre or clinic should be happy to advise you. The receptionist may be able to help you decide which therapist is the most appropriate for you or simply to help you if you want to make tentative inquiries, pick up a few leaflets and generally find out whether it's the sort of place you would like to come for treatment. Just because a practitioner works in a natural health centre doesn't guarantee they are any good, but they are likely at least to have gone through an interview system, have references, belong to a professional organization and be insured. Some centres offer a consultation with a panel of practitioners who will discuss your problem and recommend suitable therapies and therapists but this is still very rare and may be hard to find.

Computer networks are another useful source of recommendations (if you have a modem, or know someone who does), as are patient support groups, health farms and beauty treatment centres and, sometimes, public libraries, information centres and even citizens' advice bureaux.

If you can't find a natural therapist by asking around you can try contacting one of the national umbrella organizations and ask for their list of registered organizations or practitioners. Their details are listed in Appendix A. They may charge for their lists (as well as for postage and packing) and because each therapy may have several professional organizations they may ask you to specify which organization you want. If you can afford it, ask for the lot.

If you find a therapist through newspaper and magazine adverts, or *Yellow Pages*, it's a good idea to talk to them before you start treatment (see 'How to check out therapists and organizations').

---

10 ways of finding a therapist

● Word of mouth (the best method)
● Your local family medical centre
● Your local natural health centre
● Your local healthfood or alternative book shop
● Health farms and beauty treatment centres
● Local patient support groups
● National therapy organizations (but see below)
● Computer networks (you need a 'modem')
● Public libraries and information centres
● Local *Yellow Pages*, newspapers and magazines

How to check out therapists and organizations

Many therapists claim to belong to a variety of impressive-sounding organizations so it is always a very good idea to check out the background of someone you have picked from a list. This is not just because there are no set standards that apply across the board in natural therapy as there are in conventional medicine but because it is a good idea to check out anyone you know nothing about to whom you are entrusting your health (the same should really apply to choosing a family doctor). Here is a list of questions you could ask:

● When was the association founded? (Groups spring up all the time and you may find it useful to know if they have been going 50 years or started yesterday.)
● When was the therapy it represents started? (Is it ancient or some new innovation?)
● How many members does it have? (Size will give you a good idea of its public acceptance and the track record of the therapy.)
● Is it a charity or educational trust – with a proper constitution, management committee and published accounts – or is it a private limited company?

(Charities are regulated and have to operate in the public interest. Private companies don't.)

- Is it part of a larger network of professional organizations? (Groups that go their own way are on balance more suspect than those who 'join in'.)
- Does the association have a code of ethics and disciplinary procedures? If so, what are they?
- How do they assess their members? Is it linked to one particular school or college? (Be wary if the head of the association is also head of the school or college: you may be dealing with a 'one man – or woman – band'.)
- Are members covered by professional indemnity insurance against accident and malpractice?

How to check on training and qualifications

Having asked the above questions, and if you are still not sure about the experience or ability of the people listed, you may find these extra questions helpful:

- How long is the training?
- Is it full-time or part-time?
- Does it include seeing patients under supervision?
- What qualification is awarded (what do the initials after the therapist's name mean: this may be mentioned in organizations' membership lists but isn't always)
- Are the qualifications recognized?
- If so, by whom?

Making the choice

Having got as many answers as you feel you need, making your choice of therapist is really a matter of trusting your intuition. You'll know when someone suggests the right therapist for you. It's similar to that old saying

The British Medical Association's opinion

The British Medical Association recommends that anyone seeking the help of what it calls a 'non-conventional therapist' should ask the following questions:

- Is the therapist registered with a professional organization?
- Does the professional organization have:
  a public register?
  a code of practice?
  an effective disciplinary procedure and sanction?
  a complaints mechanism?
- What qualification(s) does the therapist hold?
- What training was involved in getting the qualification(s)?
- How many years has the therapist been practising?
- Is the therapist covered by professional indemnity insurance?

The BMA said that although it would like to see natural therapies regulated by law, with a single regulating body for each therapy, it did not think that all therapies needed regulating. For the majority, it said, ' the adoption of a code of practice, training structures and voluntary registration would be sufficient.'

Complementary Medicine: New Approaches to Good Practice (Oxford University Press, June 1993)

'when the pupil is ready, the master appears'. No matter how many questions you ask in the end you have to use your intuition, find someone you can trust and have a rapport with and give them a try. Your body (or mind) is asking for healing and is likely to lead you to the right therapist given the chance. Once you've made up your mind that you want healing and are willing to take responsibility for your health you will find that it is easier than you expect. You may even find that you start to feel better as soon as you have made your first appointment with the therapist. This happens surprisingly often.

What is it like seeing a natural therapist?

Seeing a natural therapist is usually easier and more straight-forward than seeing a conventional doctor. For example, many natural therapists will:

- speak to you on the 'phone themselves when you make the appointment
- give you far more time than you are used to. An initial consultation can last an hour or more. During this first visit they will ask you a lot of questions to help them understand what makes you tick and what may be the fundamental cause(s) of your problem
- charge you for their time. Some therapists offer reduced fees, and even waive fees altogether for people who genuinely cannot afford it. Some therapists who do this allocate a certain amount of 'free' or subsidised time as part of their spiritual practice (like tithing)
- will probably supply you themselves with any remedies they recommend (some, particularly homoeopaths, may even include the cost of remedies in the consultation fee).

Natural therapists come from all walks of life, from the rich to the poor, the politically left to the politically right. Two people can practise the same therapy, and be as different as chalk and cheese. You will come across as much variety in dress and behaviour as there are fashions, from the elegant and formal to the positively informal and 'woolly-haired'. Some practitioners try to look like doctors with a white coat and others are happier in jeans. A practitioners' principle method of transport may be a cadillac, Rolls Royce or bicycle.

The premises they work in reflect their attitudes to their work and the world. Some will present a 'brass plaque' image, working in a clinic with receptionist and brisk efficiency, whereas others will see you in their living room surrounded by pot-plants and domestic clutter. Image may be some indication of status but it says nothing about ability. You are as likely to find a good therapist working from home as in a clinic.

The importance of experience

'A master acupuncturist from China came to demonstrate pulse reading to a class in San Diego. The school provided a translator and a patient who had several chronic diseases, one of which was in an acute phase. The patient was brought into the lecture theatre in a wheelchair and the translator got ready to translate.

'The venerable Chinese gentleman felt the patient's pulse on the right wrist. Then he felt the pulse on the left wrist. He didn't say a word. Everyone waited. After two hours the acupuncturist said "Aaah" and put a needle into the patient – who shrieked and fainted. The acupuncturist nodded and felt the needle, like testing a cake in the oven. He checked the pulses several times and after a few minutes lifted the needle out.

'The patient opened his eyes, said the pain in his shoulders had gone, the pain in his back had gone and his head felt fine. He tested the weight on his feet and found he could stand up. He said "I feel great," and walked out of the room.

'The elderly acupuncturist said something in Chinese and the translator translated: "To read pulses takes much practice and much patience".'

The American healer Jessica Macbeth (now living in Britain) tells the above story in her training courses, but it is relevant for anyone who wants to understand any form of natural medicine. It illustrates two very important points:
● It takes time and patience to become a 'master'.
● Anyone can become a natural therapist, but it takes a life time of experience to be able to do it with the minimum of effort for maximum result.

This is the main reason why natural medicine isn't more widespread. It takes time and patience to do it exceptionally well. In a society that demands instant results time and patience are rare commodities.

The more experienced the therapist the more skilled they are likely to be. The matter of experience is very important. If an acupuncturist has spent a lifetime feeling pulses, making his or her diagnosis and using acupuncture, he or she will be able to help you more easily than the most highly-qualified Western doctor who has learned a little acupuncture in weekend courses. In every field of medicine there are people who are the equivalent of consultants. In natural medicine these are the acupuncturists, homoeopaths, healers and other practitioners that other therapists turn to for advice and training. So it's always a good idea to go to the most experienced practitioner you can find.

Experienced or not, though, make sure the therapist you choose is qualified, insured and a member of a professional body. In some states in the USA they must also be in possession of a legal licence to practise.

Sensible precautions

- Don't pay out in advance for any treatment unless it is specifically for medicines or tests needing a 'down payment'. Even this is rare and no ethical practitioner will ask for fees in advance.
- Don't listen to anyone who 'guarantees' you a cure. It's impossible.
- Don't stop taking drugs prescribed by your family doctor on a therapist's say-so without first talking the matter over with your doctor. There may be a good reason why stopping suddenly or without preparation is dangerous and a good natural therapist will know this.
- Don't see a male therapist on your own if you are

female and feel nervous about it. Feel free to have a friend present if you need to undress and you are happier this way.

● Don't hesitate to cancel an appointment (or not to book another) if you don't like the therapist, the place or the treatment. If you cancel remember to try and give at least 24 hours notice or the therapist may charge you. Ask as many questions as you like.

What to do if things go wrong

The most important thing to decide is whether you think the therapist has done his or her absolute best to get you better without hurting or harming you in any way. Failure to cure you is not an offence and they are probably as disappointed about it as you are. But failure to take proper care and treat you with professional respect is both offensive and a professional offence. If this should happen to you the first step is to complain to the therapist.

If this doesn't work contact the professional body to which the therapist belongs. In the US, complain to the appropriate licensing body. If you feel the therapist's behaviour is the result of something either incompetent or unethical report them to their professional body and go elsewhere. You may also want to write to them to tell them how you feel about what they have done. They need to know that what they have done is wrong so that they do not repeat the offence.

In some countries, such as Britain, natural medicine has few controls – which gives both freedom and responsibilities. It means there is little or no professional comeback if therapists behave unprofessionally or irresponsibly. In Britain, for example, practitioners are not obliged to join a professional organization, and the professional organizations themselves have little or no real power to discipline members who break the rules. Expelled practitioners are still free to practise under UK law provided they don't break any civil or criminal law. In the US the regulations vary from state to state. Find out what the local regulations are.

In reality, bad reputations are bad for business and therapists with bad reputations tend to go out of business very quickly. If you are not happy or satisfied with your treatment or the therapist's behaviour, change your therapist and tell everyone why you switched. If the therapist works at a natural health centre, it's particularly important to tell them about your decision. They will not want their reputation tarnished by an unprofessional practitioner.

In conclusion: Marion's story

It's just as well that natural therapists are so varied. It makes it more likely that you will find someone who can help you and your migraine. It is important to find someone who you feel happy with, someone who can help you to help yourself. Many people are lucky enough to find a therapist they can trust with all their health problems.

The important thing is not to expect miracles. You may be lucky and find the answer to your migraine very quickly or you may need a great deal of patience and end up by using several approaches – like Marion:

'My father had migraine, but not very often. My mother referred to them as 'dad's bilious turns' and they frightened me as a child, hearing him retching and being sick. My earliest memory of my own migraines was when I was at college in the sixties. I changed my lifestyle, environment and diet. I drank coffee for the first time in my life and I didn't allow myself much relaxation. My father didn't want me to go to college or have a career and I was over-conscientious, trying to prove myself. About a year before going to college I was involved in a road accident and that might have had an effect because my family doctor gave me manipulation and that gave me temporary relief.

'I had about ten weekly sessions of acupuncture, which helped to "balance" my energy but didn't give much relief in the long-term. I tried homoeopathy, tissue salts and other remedies. But I took them without advice or much knowledge so they were not much help. I found the things that really helped me were moving to Cornwall, stopping teaching, being more contented and happier with myself, cranial osteopathy, adopting an anti-candida diet, having regular meals, massage, doing relaxation, the Alexander Technique, drinking plenty of water and taking large doses of vitamin C. I think all those things have helped – and although I've had headaches I haven't had a real blinder of a migraine for years – MARION G.

Many people who suffer from migraine will identify with Marion's experience, and admire her perseverance, which seems to be an essential part of getting well. Just as migraine may be caused by many different factors you may need to turn to many different therapies before you can say goodbye to your migraine. On the other hand, you may find that a single, simple remedy does the trick instantly:

'I was cured as soon as I learned how to meditate. I didn't have a headache, let alone a migraine.'
– ANDREW F.

'I came off chocolate and dairy products and the migraines disappeared just like that. It was remarkable' – HOWARD H.

'I must have had four migraines a year for years, but each time it's always a tremendous surprise. Last year I felt one coming up but I diverted it by cancelling appointments and I've not had one for several years' – SHEILAH S.

'It's such a relief to have conquered my migraines' – JEAN S.

If they can cure their migraines so can you – the natural way.

APPENDIX A

Useful organizations

The following listing of organizations is for information only and does not imply any endorsement, nor do the organizations listed necessarily agree with the views expressed in this book.

INTERNATIONAL

International Federation of Practitioners of Natural Therapeutics
46 Pulens Crescent
Sheet
Petersfield
Hampshire GU31 4DH, UK.
Tel 730 266 790
Fax 730 260 058.

AUSTRALASIA

Australian Brain Foundation
746 Burke Road
Camberwell 3124
Victoria, Australia.
Tel 038 822 203.

Australian Migraine Association
PO Box 2504
Kent Town Centre
South Australia 5071.

Australian Natural Therapists Association
PO Box 308
Melrose Park
South Australia 5039.
Tel 8297 9533
Fax 8297 0003.

Australian Traditional Medicine Society
PO Box 442 *or*
Suite 3, First Floor,
120 Blaxland Road
Ryde
New South Wales 2112.
Australia
Tel 2808 2825
Fax 2809 7570

The Headache Clinic
Royal Brisbane Hospital
Herston Road
Herston
Queensland 4006.

**New Zealand Natural Health
Practitioners Accreditation
Board**
Po Box 37-491
Auckland, New Zealand.
Tel 9625 9966.

NORTH AMERICA

**American Association of
Naturopathic Physicians**
2800 East Madison Street,
Suite 200
Seattle
Washington 98112, USA
or
PO Box 20386
Seattle
Washington 98102, USA.
Tel 206 323 7610
Fax 206 323 7612.

**American Holistic Medical
Association**
4101 Lake Boone Trail, Suite 201
Raleigh
North Carolina 27607, USA.
Tel 919 787 5146
Fax 919 787 4916.

**American Academy of Medical
Preventics**
6151 West Century Boulevard,
Suite 1114
Los Angeles
California 90045, USA.
Tel 213 645 5350.

**Canadian Holistic Medical
Association**
700 Bay Street
PO Box 101, Suite 604

Toronto
Ontario M5G 1Z6, Canada.
Tel 416 599 0447.

National Headache Foundation
5252 North Western Avenue
Chicago
Illinois 60625, USA.
Tel (in Illinois) 1-800-523-8858
(outside Illinois) 1-800-843-2256.

Migraine Foundation of Canada
390 Brunswick Avenue
Toronto
Ontario M5R 224, Canada.
Tel 416 920 4916

**Scripps Clinic and Research
Foundation**
10666 North Torrey Pines Road
La Jolla
Ca 92037, USA.

SOUTHERN AFRICA

**South African Homoeopaths,
Chiropractors & Allied
Professions Board**
PO Box 17055
0027 Gooenkloof
South Africa.
Tel 2712 466 455.

UK

**British Complementary
Medicine Association**
St Charles Hospital
Exmoor Street
London W10 6BZ.
Tel 081 964 1205
Fax 081 964 1207.

Council for Complementary &
Alternative Medicine
179 Gloucester Place
London NW1 6DX.
Tel 071 724 9103
Fax 071 724 5330.

British Migraine Association
178a High Road
Byfleet
Surrey KT14 7ED.
Tel 0932 352468

Institute for Complementary
Medicine
P.O. Box 194
London SE16 1QZ
Tel 071 237 5165
Fax 071 237 5175.

City of London Migraine Clinic
22 Charterhouse Square
London EC1M 6DX.
Tel 071-251 3322.

Useful further reading

Migraine, Oliver Sacks (Picador, UK, 1993). A classic.

Overcoming Migraine, Betsy Wycoff (Station Hill Press, USA, 1991). A guide to treatment and prevention.

The Migraine Handbook, Jenny Lewis with the British Migraine Association (Vermilion, UK, 1993).

Coping Successfully with Migraine, Sue Dyson (Sheldon Press, UK, 1991). City of London Migraine Clinic cases.

Mind-Body Medicine: How to Use Your Mind for Better Health, ed Daniel Goleman & Joel Courin (Consumers Reports Books, USA, 1993)

Raw Energy, Leslie and Susannah Kenton (Arrow Books, UK, 1989)

Mega-Nutrition, Richard Kunin (New American Library, USA, 1981)

Thorsons Introductory Guide to Kinesiology, Maggie La Tourelle and Anthea Courtenay (Thorsons, UK, 1992).

Migraine: Special Diet Cookbook, Celia Norman (Thorsons, UK, 1990)

Food Combining for Health,
Doris Grant and Jean Joice (Thorsons, UK, 1984)

Moon Over Water, Jessica Macbeth (Gateway, UK, 1990)

Acupuncture Energy-Balancing for Body, Mind and Spirit, Peter Mole (Element, UK, 1993)

Homoeopathy: Medicine of the New Man, George Vithoulkas (Thorsons, UK, 1985)

Thorsons Introductory Guide to Healing, Eileen Herzberg (Thorsons, UK, 1988).

Sun Over Mountain, Jessica Macbeth (Gateway Books, UK, 1991).

Book of Stress Survival: How to Relax and De-stress Your Life, Alix Kirsta (Unwin, UK, 1986)

Pressure at Work: A Survival Guide, Tanya Arroba, Kim Jones (McGraw Hill, UK, 1987)

Stress Protection Plan: How to Stay Healthy Under Pressure, Leon Chaitow (Thorsons, UK, 1992)

Index